SHERWIN B. NULAND

SIMON & SCHUSTER
NEW YORK LONDON SYDNEY SINGAPORE

The
Mysteries
Within

A SURGEON
REFLECTS ON
MEDICAL MYTHS

SIMON & SCHUSTER
Rockefeller Center
1230 Avenue of the Americas
New York, NY 10020

Designed by Karolina Harris

Manufactured in the United States of America

10 9 8 7 6 5 4 3 2 1

Library of Congress Cataloging-in-Publication Data

Nuland, Sherwin B.
     The mysteries within : a surgeon reflects on medical myths / Sherwin
B. Nuland.
          p.   cm.
          1. Body, Human—Folklore.   2. Body, Human—Mythology.
3. Human anatomy—Mythology.   4. Body, Human—Symbolic aspects.
I. Title.
R133.N77 2000
610—dc21   99-088659

     ISBN 0-684-85486-4

Acknowledgments

THE operating room is a storyteller's place. Of course, the newest gossip is heard there and the oldest jokes—but those are not the stories I mean. I refer instead to the tales of surgery—of remembered patients, of diseases obscure and common, of unusual situations encountered, difficulties overcome and difficulties sometimes not overcome. And I refer also to stories of the long-gone past, because surgeons, of all medical specialists, seem most to honor the history of their art.

And there are stories, too, of individual organs: their behavior normal and abnormal; the characteristics that make operating on them either easy or difficult; and the legends that have been associated with them through the ages. Stories of then and now are the lore of surgery. They are the tradition that we elders pass on to those who will follow us.

Beginning with my medical-school days, I have been hearing and telling these legendary tales for almost half a century. I was fortunate to serve my clinical apprenticeship in an atmosphere where the heritage of surgery and its modern-day fascinations was deemed to be the patrimony of every novitiate privileged to join our ever-expanding clan. I spent thousands of hours in the operating room with some master storytellers, and nowadays my own best tales are often improved by new information provided by young colleagues. I have had many teachers, and still do.

Attempting to acknowledge all the contributors to a gradual process is a slippery proposition at best, doomed to incompleteness. Who can remember, and why should a reader care? But certain names must be mentioned. There are three men who carried me into the excitement of medical lore at the same time they were carrying me—as though in a troika—into the excitement of the surgical life itself. They are all still living, and this in itself reassures me that my sustenance has not yet left me. One of them is in his nineties, and the other two are in their mid-eighties. They are Gustaf Lindskog, Mark Hayes, and William Glenn, my teachers and my friends.

It should by now be apparent that I have been gathering the material in this book for a long time—fifty years, in fact. During the middle period of that time, I formed deep friendships with several men and women, all a decade or more older than I, whose effect on my life was unexpected and quite remarkable, especially since it occurred when I was in my forties. I had known several of them for long periods before our closeness developed, but the others were new to me. In their own individual ways, each of them thought I was a better man than I really am, and I had no choice but to be as they thought me. In the broadest sense, they became my collective Muse. It is to their memories that this book is dedicated.

The preceding paragraphs are by way of explaining how I came to write this book. Unknowingly, I have been preparing for it all these decades. No matter the gradual nature of their aggregation, the time came that the stories had to go beyond being told. They were demanding to be written down. And for the completion of that absorbing task I am indebted to still other friends, who have shared countless hours of talk with me, and helped to redefine again and again my perceptions of the past and of the present. Enfolded into the chapters of this book are notions that came clear during long conversations with Joseph Fruton, Ferenc Gyorgyey, Jay Katz, and Robert Massey. Joe has, in addition, led me toward the clear, brilliant light of dispassionate science; Ferenc has led me toward centuries of sources and their interpretation; Jay has led me toward insights into the human condition, and my own; and Bob has led me toward the *humanitas* inherent in the art of healing. As in the past, Bob has read every page of this book's manuscript. He has corrected my wandering, and at several points kept me from making a complete ass of myself. Like Joe and Ferenc and Jay, he has never hesitated to challenge my assumptions, and more than once found them faulty.

I am indebted also to other friends, who knowledgeably provided answers to the many questions that came up during the course of writing, and knew just how to find whatever it was that I was looking for at various junctures. They are Toby Appel, James Boyer, Richard Eisenberg, Worth Estes, Jan Glover, David Henry Kagan, Bernard Lytton, Wayne Meeks, Akiva Northern, James Ponet, Heinrich von Staden, and Barry Zaret.

Luck plays a part, and in my case luck takes the form of having had my work fall into the hands of skilled editors. For the artistry of Bob Bender, I feel not only gratitude but even a kind of awe at his wise and gentle touch, not to mention his support. David Rosenthal, Simon & Schuster's publisher, has energized this project with the enthusiasm he added to it from the start, which has kept my own optimisms at their highest.

There are agents and there are literary agents—and then there are book people who represent authors because they admire them and because they love literature. I have been endowed with two such, who entered my life with a phone call in 1991 and have from that day understood not only what it is that this surgeon needed to do as a writer but as a man, too, and as the father of a family. Glen Hartley and Lynn Chu have been my guides through the labyrinths of the publishing world, in which I would surely have lost my way without them. The word "guide" derives from an Indo-European source meaning "to see" or "to have vision." Nothing more need be said.

As for vision—for her sight, insight, foresight, and an image of her husband that is far more realistic than his own, I would dedicate every word I write to Sarah Peterson Nuland if I could. Instead, I dedicate my life.

I have had Muses—and they are with me still.
Arthur Chiel
David Clement
Thomas Forbes
Grace Goldin
Madeline Stanton
and especially Elizabeth Thomson

CONTENTS

INTRODUCTION

EACH of our internal organs has a personality of its own, and a mythology too. Any surgeon will tell you that, but even surgeons know only a small percentage of the stories that have shaped the image of one or another of the structures they fondle daily in the name of healing.

Long before physicians had so much as made a start toward any valid understanding of human anatomy, rumors abounded over just what it is that goes on beneath the layers of skin, fat, and fiber hiding the inner man from his own direct scrutiny.* Sounds were heard, rumblings were felt, and it must often have seemed to our earliest forebear that autonomous lives were being lived in the capacious cavities of his body. Through the slaughter of beasts and of his enemies, he knew that inside of him dwelt structures of various shapes, colors, and consistencies. Some of them continued to wriggle or pulsate for seconds

---

*Throughout this book I use "man," "he," and "his" in the generic sense, to refer to both men and women.

or minutes after a chest or an abdomen had been laid open with primitive weapons. To our ancient ancestors, life was movement. If an organ moved in the depths of their bodies, perhaps it had a life of its own. Perhaps there were animals within. At the very least, there was mystery.

That notion took tens of millennia to fade from the minds of humanity, as people developed cultures and societies, and began to live together in villages and then cities. Meanwhile, it came to be thought that certain of the organs determined the character of some of the qualities in a man's nature, such as intellect and mood. Like so many other peoples, the Egyptians believed that the larger structures were creatures with whims of their own, migrating where they wished from neck to pelvis. Such fantastical notions did not entirely disappear even when societies reached a high level of sophistication and rational philosophies of man's existence came into being. Not unexpectedly, the sex organs were the last to lose the reputation of being independent. When Plato called the uterus "an animal within an animal," he was not speaking metaphorically. Echoing a common belief of his time, he was convinced that under proper conditions it "becomes seriously angry and moves all over the body."

From such shrouded and uncertain beginnings, an entire body (and the word is here used advisedly) of mythology and legend gradually developed, in which every organ ultimately became surrounded with superstitions, fanciful stories, and real events involving real people. Whatever the viscus, a singular personal history exists for it. Century after century—slowing almost to a halt during the Middle Ages but accelerating with the late Renaissance—new knowledge was brought forward, and new bits of narrative were added to the lore. Also, new investigators entered the arena. Once science came onto the scene in the sixteenth and seventeenth centuries, the mystically perceived personalities of the various viscera began to take on a more well-defined form, molded from the experiences and observations— and in some cases, exploits—of an ever-enlarging corps of highly individualistic personalities. Not only physicians but soldiers, storytellers, poets, and adventurers of every sort were quick to comment on the tubular or solid, firm or soft, moving or still, undulating or pulsating viabilities they were becoming familiar with at the bedside, in autopsy rooms, and at scenes of carnage.

Even when made by scientists, the commentary was not always scientific. There was often a colorful subjectivity about it—even a note of wishful thinking, awe, or perhaps fear or warning. An organ's legend is the sum of the accumulated memories that have become associated with it. The memories, the recorded history, and our present scientifically obtained knowledge form the basis upon which to understand that organ's personality. Beginning perhaps with the mystical musings of a Babylonian or Egyptian priest and ending in the ultramicroscopic manifestations of today's shamans of molecular medicine, the legend is imbedded with the stories of the people who are the witnesses to its details. They are that legend's creators.

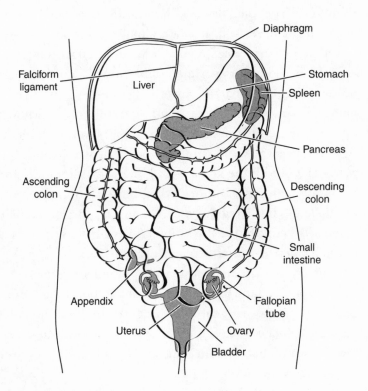

The organs of the abdomen.

Whether a discovery, military battle, interpersonal conflict, intellectual current, or simply one of the myriad daily occurrences that chron-
icle the course of centuries of development, each event in the
cavalcade of a growing legend comes from the annals of someone's
life. Whatever else it may be, the legend surrounding an organ is a tale
of the individual men and women who have added bits and pieces to
the whole. It is permeated with their humanity. Be the fragments of
the narrative harrowing scenes in the operating room, tales of discovery in deprived or opulent surroundings, the result of serendipity, of
chance, of competitiveness, of collaboration, or even of error—or
perhaps the issue of an obsessed seeker's determined quest—they are
the stuff of human experience; they are the expression of mankind's
nature.

It is also mankind's nature to cling to myths even when new information reveals their basis to be, in fact, nothing more than the fabled
storytelling of a people. Science has never completely replaced
mythology, and it never will. Instead, alongside the knowledge that
can be validated by evidence acceptable to an intellect trained in the
dispassionate methods of experiment and induction, there seems always to flow a parallel stream of unverifiable perceptions. Such a system of alternate varieties of understanding fulfills, in its own way, the
need for mystery that has always permeated all levels of human consciousness. It preserves what might be thought of as a demotic form of
biology, associated with the kitchen-wisdom of grandmothers and the
notions of all manner of unorthodox healers. Superstition, too,
abounds. Folktales involving the viscera being as old as humankind itself, we cling like children to their familiar rhythms, sometimes allowing them to influence our perceptions of reality.

The tendency toward mysticism is ingrained in human nature.
Superstition, religion, and medicine have made their long journey together, and even now are unable to let go of one another's hands.
Religion is the reluctant fellow traveler of superstition, and science attempts to disown them both—in vain. The links joining the three are
indissoluble. They will never be destroyed.

Even after the so-called scientific revolution of the seventeenth century, researchers imbued their theories of the body with the superstitious and also the religious beliefs that permeated the thinking of all people of the time. The new discoveries in human biology, in particular, were interpreted in such a way that they fit into the perspective of Church dogma. Even by the most astute minds, spiritual forces were thought to actuate the functioning of organs; the soul and Divine Will were seen in the behavior of all living things; supernatural causes were invoked to explain what was not yet understood. But in doing this, the scientists and churchmen hid their eyes, refusing to see that they were merely following in the same path that had always been trod since men first looked up at the skies and attributed everything in nature to celestial influences. The great teachers of classical Greece had been no exception. While seeking wisdom in nature stripped of supernature, they nevertheless succumbed to the human predisposition to see the basis of life in preconceived patterns, in their case based on entire philosophies of the universe that they had no way of confirming. Though not called religion, theirs was a religion of its own; though not called superstition, theirs was a superstition of its own.

The history of modern biomedicine—and modern science, too—is the history of man's diminishing need to fill the gaps in his understanding of nature by resorting to the mystical, whether in the form of magic or through the teachings of philosophy or the Church. In thus separating himself, he has had to take leave of precious reassurances that he can control his destiny by appealing to higher power in moment-to-moment aspects of his life. He has had to reject—at least when interpreting scientific evidence—any possibility that there is some greater purpose guiding the universe and his life. Such a departure from eons-long certainty is frightening, and in any event not totally possible. For there is that in each of us which craves the mystery we have with such difficulty tried to abandon in our thirst for detached scientific knowledge. And there is another craving too, related to the first in that it is a form of magical thinking: Like the child that each of us remains, we have preconceptions of what is real and interpret all that we see through the lens of our own desires and fears. A thing is so because we ordain it to be so; we can make things happen by ordaining that they happen. In the subterranean depths of our inchoate expectations of how the world works, we hear the old refrain, "Wishing will make it so."

All of this was expressed aphoristically by Claude Bernard, the great French scientist of the mid-nineteenth century, who is appropriately considered to be the father of modern physiology. Bernard devoted considerable thought to the personal characteristics required to do dispassionate research, and decided that the kind of reasoning needed for the purpose does not exist as an innate quality of the human mind. Here is how he summed it all up, in 1865: "Man is by nature metaphysical and arrogant. Accordingly, he thinks that the idealistic creations of his mind, which correspond to his feelings, are identical with reality. From this it follows that the experimental method is not really natural to him, and that only after lengthy wanderings in theological and scholastic discussion has he recognized at last the sterility of his efforts in this direction."

This book is not an attack on religion. Far from it. But it is a testament to its author's unshakable conviction that religion and science do not mix well. Only natural means can be used to explain natural phenomena. Only a mind imbued with faith can comprehend the wonders of faith. But true religious faith is not superstition, and it is certainly not magic.

The first healers were indeed magicians, and even today doctors are magicians of a sort, though they deny the role that mysticism plays in their authority, and even in their power to heal. They are heir to a millennia-old tradition in which confidence in their ability and acceptance of their authority have been useful in healing. They are heir to mythologies which can on the one hand be employed in their therapies or on the other may subvert their attempts at cure.

These mythologies take on different forms, resulting in practices as harmless as saying "gesundheit" when someone sneezes, all along the spectrum of increasing danger to such counterproductive behaviors as refusing medical treatment in order to seek guidance from questionable sources or quacks. Every system of what is called traditional medicine finds its origins in the lore associated with the organs of the body, having remarkable similarities in all societies. Because some of the lore is based on accurate understanding obtained through centuries of observation, it has real value; because some of it, like so much New Age belief, is the result of unfocused thought, misinterpreted experience, or downright fraud, it is not only unhelpful but may do serious harm. The role of millennia of mythology is stronger in our everyday thinking than most of us realize.

The purpose of this book is to explore the journey that superstition, religion, and medicine have taken in one another's company. Having considered the various ways in which such an exploration might be most pleasurably conducted—both for readers and myself—I elected to choose a group of internal organs with which I have become very familiar through the years of my surgical career and to use them as examples of what mankind experienced during our travels toward modern thought. What I have done for each organ is to trace from earliest times the ways in which it—stomach, liver, spleen, heart, and uterus—was understood by physicians and the laity of every era, until biomedical science finally elucidated its most minute workings. As an extension of the story of the uterus, I have added a chapter on the evolution of knowledge of reproduction. Each of these chronicles begins in myth and ends in modernity.

These are stories about the evolution of specifically Western thought. Though evidence abounds of the historic influence of certain Eastern concepts and of similarities in some of our mystical notions with tribal healing beliefs in various areas of the world, I have restricted myself to one more or less direct line. It stretches from earliest humans to the Fertile Crescent where our civilization began, and then on to the formulations of the ancient Egyptians and Greeks, before eventually reaching the modern cultures of which we are a part.

As in past writings, I have not been able to resist telling the stories of certain of my own most unforgettable experiences with these organs. (All but one, that is. Absent is a tale of the uterus because I have had less personal contact with its clinical behavior than with the others.) My fascination with medicine has been renewed over and over again by challenging and exhilarating contacts with patients, disease, and the response of the organs of the body that I have come to know so well. In writing this book, it has seemed to me that an enjoyable introduction to the narrative of each organ's journey through superstition and science might be a case history taken from the annals of my own encounters with it. Perhaps in doing this I have indulged myself just a bit, but the storytelling has added immeasurably to what was for me already an immensely gratifying re-creation of these voyages. I can only hope that readers will find as much pleasure in reading about these memorable events as I have had in recalling them.

CHAPTER ONE

THE STOMACH:

A LITTLE BOY'S

BIG SECRET

No matter how often a surgeon performs the same operation, it is different each time. Any operating room nurse can tell you that. The sequential precision of predictable steps so exactingly depicted in manuals of surgical technique resembles the real thing about as much as a diagram of human anatomy looks like a human being.

To take something simple: Of the many hundreds of appendectomies I have done during a career of thirty-five years, no two were the same. Even such a straightforward operative procedure for a straightforward disease, divisible into a short series of straightforward technical maneuvers that were standardized almost one hundred years ago, done by an operator of long experience—even under such circumstances every case is a novelty. And some of those novelties can be daunting tests of skill and confidence.

On bedside rounds one day during the period of my training, the senior attending surgeon, a man highly respected for his dexterity and judgment, was asked to name the half-dozen most difficult operative cases he had encountered in his career. After a moment's thought, he replied that three of them had been appendectomies. His answer surprised no one in the group of interns and residents who were crowded around him. In the few years of our embryonic surgical experience, every one of us had already seen enough to appreciate what he meant.

Although the configurations of human innards do not vary nearly as much as do those of our outards (a word that exists in no dictionary, but should), they nevertheless reveal unmistakable variations among individuals—and only surgeons ever find out about them. The way in which an organ is attached by ligaments and folds of tissue to its surroundings, for example, is in general predictable, and yet just enough personal difference occurs that an operator never knows beforehand whether the viscus he is approaching will come up easily into his seeking hands or require deep dissection to free it. Friend appendix, in fact, epitomizes this kind of anatomical uncertainty. Being attached to the large intestine only at one narrow end of its wormlike body, the appendix is free to turn upward toward the liver, downward toward the pelvis, sideward toward the center of the abdomen, forward toward the abdominal wall, or even retrocecal, which means it has tucked itself up behind the bowel into a hidden location. The appendix may be as short as a stumpy inch or as willowy as five or six times that length. There is no telling where its tip may be found. Other organs, though not as variable, have unpredictabilities of their own.

And then there is the problem of fat. The copiousness of the cushions of fatty tissue lying between internal structures depends in general on an individual's station along the spectrum between leanness and obesity. Thin people are a great deal easier to operate upon than are the chubbies, who hide vital structures deep within thick, greasy blankets of adiposity. Among those concealed vital structures are blood vessels, which have an obnoxious tendency to make uncharted course changes now and then, obstinately refusing to reach their destination via the route assigned to them by anatomy books. Lying in wait for the unwary, or perhaps lurking within a fatty bolster, an unanticipated artery or vein—and nerves are known to do this too—can affect the entire plan of a surgeon's work, and sometimes its outcome.

Beyond even these considerations, the occasional occurrence of a congenital variation of structure must be taken into account. The operating team always has to be on guard for such an abnormality, especially because it may involve blood vessels or the slender ducts that carry secretions and other vital fluids to their destinations. Some of these inborn irregularities can present major challenges, or at least major surprises. From time to time, for example, one or another viscus or a part of it must be sought in an area of the body where it seems not to belong. I am not at all unique among surgeons to have removed thyroid tissue from the chest, found the right colon on the left side of the abdomen, and taken an ovary or appendix out of a hernia bulging into the uppermost part of the thigh.

All of these are strictly anatomical variations, but it is the evolution of the patient's disease that is the greatest determinant of the differing conditions that must be dealt with at operation. Some pathologies will enlarge an organ, and some will shrink it or leave its size unchanged; some will be diagnosed before they involve surrounding tissues sufficiently to make dissection hazardous, and some will be found to be so far advanced as to require major modifications in the planned operative approach.

Diseases may attack an organ in any of an array of ways—one manifestation of pathology might originate in the structure's center and another at its periphery; associated blood vessels may be attacked early or late in the course of a sickness; some diseases (such as those that increase hormone production to toxic levels) require the gentlest and most painstaking of surgical approaches lest even minimal manipulation or pressure force the release of large amounts of noxious substance into the bloodstream; others (such as a ruptured aorta) resemble a scene of carnage, and demand extremely rapid, forceful, and sometimes inelegant maneuvers to bring a life-threatening situation under control.

Although a patient's basic anatomy and disease account for the great majority of the variation from one surgical undertaking to another, there are still other factors, which, though their effect is less, can sometimes carry great significance during a person's hours on the operating table. The quality of the anesthesia, the experience of the team, and the patient's general health are examples, but there are others to consider. Like the rest of humanity, surgeons tend to be unduly influenced by their most recent experiences. Even an operator who has done a particular procedure many times may at short notice decide to change one or another aspect of his accustomed approach because of something that happened while working on his last patient; or perhaps he has heard a lecture on the topic during the medical conference from which he has just returned. Occasionally a last-minute corridor conversation or a chat in the scrub room may make him choose to alter his plan. Time of day, level of fatigue—even the state of domestic tranquillity he left at home that morning—all of these have an effect on every member of the team, and sometimes make an operation unforgettable when it might otherwise have been easily filed away in the part of a surgeon's memory reserved for the ordinary.

I have been referring here to operations done with relative frequency. For the reasons given or others, some cases will be so unusual that they stand out in a surgeon's mind for the rest of his life. But in addition to that list, there exists a special category within even less commonly done procedures—these are the real *rarae aves*. By this I mean the one-and-onlies. These are the operations of such a unique type that the members of the team will regale one another with their details when they meet at reunions or conventions decades later, even in far-flung parts of the world. Some of these procedures are firsts, or at least firsts in a given hospital—the first organ transplant, the first use of the heart-lung machine, the first video-controlled gallbladder operation—but some are memorable because no member of the team has ever seen their like before or since. Like all surgeons, I have a few of those once-in-a-lifetime adventures tucked away in the back of my mind, ready to be pulled out and relived at a moment's notice.

One of them involves the stomach.

MY patient had been an independent citizen for all of six weeks, the first two of which were spent in the preemie unit of the Yale–New

Haven Hospital. Although he was born only nine days before the anticipated time, his birth weight of 2055 grams, or about $4\frac{1}{2}$ pounds, was well short of the criterion then considered to be the lower limit of normal.

My operation on little Clyde Greene Jr., as I'll call him, took place almost forty years ago, but the condition for which it was done was so singular that the details of his hospitalization are easily recalled. Just to be sure, I verified them by having the hospital's record room dig out the child's chart. Reading through those old pages made it all seem like yesterday.

Clyde Jr. was brought to the emergency room by his parents, with a history of having been vomiting in projectile fashion after most feedings for the previous three days. But it was not the vomiting that was on his eighteen-year-old mother's mind. After all, she explained to the admitting nurse, the baby had done the same during his first few days of life, and it had stopped spontaneously. What worried her was that he had begun to have diarrhea twenty-four hours earlier. It was this new problem that had prompted the trip to the hospital from the parents' home in Branford, a typical old New England shoreline town a few miles east of New Haven.

As a social worker would later discover, the house in which the Greenes lived was not in fact their own. The young couple were lodging with Clyde Sr.'s sister, her husband, and their two children, as well as two other in-laws. All told, there were six adults and three children in the crowded five-room home. Whether the reason for the living arrangements was Clyde Sr.'s weekly income of only sixty-three dollars as a lumberyard worker or, as the social worker would later conclude, "that they were rather fearful of setting up an independent household," the younger Greenes had been living this way since moving to Branford from rural Maine about six months earlier.

When examined by the pediatric intern on emergency room duty, Clyde Jr. was found to look remarkably healthy, although a bit dehydrated and still small for his age. His skin tone was reasonably good, weight was up to seven pounds ten and a half ounces, and he seemed in general like an active, healthy child—healthy that is, with the exception of his belly, which was markedly distended. Not only was it distended, but the intern and others who later examined the baby thought they could feel a rather large, firm mass in its upper region, just below the rib cage. Manual pressure through the abdominal wall on this poorly defined structure did not seem to cause the baby any discomfort. No one, from the chief resident in pediatrics on down, could come up with a diagnosis that might explain the presence of a big, solid lump in the belly of a six-week-old undersized kid.

The most dependable of emergency room procedures was now called upon, a protocol universally acknowledged to be without peer when the team is faced with an inscrutable diagnostic dilemma: call a consultant and order an X ray. Since the child was not being admitted as a private patient of one of the senior staff, his care fell to the young doctors doing their specialty training. This is how it came about that I, in my final year of residency before being set loose on the world as what is euphemistically called "a fully qualified surgeon," came to be the consultant.

It is no secret that pediatricians and internists like to think of themselves as more knowledgeable and cleverer by far than surgeons. They refer to their work as "cognitive" to distinguish it from ours, which they prefer to see as merely "technical"—or even worse, "manual." Not surprisingly then, a surgeon (particularly a young and incompletely formed one), when called to consult on a case that is baffling colleagues in a specialty whose members consider themselves to exist on a higher mental plane than his, is provided with a highly valued opportunity to strut. Characteristically, he will enter the arena in his most oracular mode; the anticipation of a triumph over smugness breeds a certain heady self-assurance. I was hardly an exception.

As I strode toward the emergency room in answer to my page, I mused with more than a small degree of satisfaction on the mixed emotions that predictably awaited my arrival there. On the one hand, by dint of the very fact of requesting a consultation, the pediatricians were being forced into acknowledging their need for diagnostic help. Worse yet, having to seek such help from a surgeon—of all possible sources, *a surgeon*—is tantamount to a frank confession of failure; to the tender psyche of the pediatricians it means being supplicant to a form of life beneath them. On the other hand, there did remain the possibility—the hope, even—that the surgeon whose intellectual endowments they derided would prove to be the vehicle by which the sick child for whom they had been given responsibility would get the treatment he needed. In other words, the surgeon might—just might—come up with the correct diagnosis and be able to help the kid.

And yet, it is not within a pediatrician's or internist's worldview that surgeons should, even on occasion, display more formidable diagnostic skills than members of their own more cerebrally oriented specialties. It is their unshakable conviction that our proper role in the community of physicians is to act only on their advice. Were they to choose, we would cut only on dotted lines of their design. This is an intramural battle that began in the Renaissance. Today still taken with just enough seriousness, it keeps the competitive fires burning ever brightly. Fortunately for patients and doctors alike, the energy expended in feeding the flames is more often the source of increased illumination than of hot air.

With this background, no surgeon can be blamed if he sees such a diagnostic consultation as the opportunity for a real coup, whose idealized fulfillment has him appearing dramatically at the bedside, placing an ostentatiously gentle hand on the belly, finding something that has been overlooked by all previous examiners, and triumphantly declaring his (obviously correct and obviously brilliant) diagnosis: some pathology that has eluded one and all until his luminescent arrival. The perfect scenario would then have him go on to describe his planned operation to the humbled physicians who had called him and the suitably impressed patient he is about to rescue, whom he then personally wheels off to the operating room for the implementation of the grand plan. The entire sequence of events is a proclamation of authority. Every surgeon longs for such moments.

I was riding a brief wave of success that morning, having only a few days earlier scored on the pediatricians by correctly diagnosing a condition known as Meckel's diverticulitis in a ten-month-old, for whom they had complacently called me to do an operation for what they presumed to be a form of intestinal obstruction called intussusception. The baby's disease was an example of one of those rare times when hoofbeats heard under one's window turn out to be caused by a passing zebra rather than the expected horse, and I was rather puffed up over having found a tiny clue that had made the distinction. That I had accidentally stumbled on it by dumb luck did not at all lessen the high regard in which I was still holding myself. The certainty that I was heading toward another competitive bull's-eye was in the forefront of my thoughts as I approached the examining room where my prospective patient awaited me. I could not have been more absorbed by the aura in which I felt myself to be strutting.

Trying to hide my smugness, I listened with seemly patience as the pediatric intern deferentially presented the case history to me. At the conclusion of that formality, I stepped—with the air of command that comes so easily to surgeons—into the examining room, exuding the self-assurance I felt. After inspecting the baby with a long, careful look, I lightly laid the flat of my stethoscope on his bloated abdomen and listened for a long minute. Not hearing anything abnormal, I proceeded with certitude to the ultimate weapon in my diagnostic panoply: I laid a hand on the belly. The definitive moment had arrived.

The abdominal wall itself was soft, and the baby did not seem bothered by the gradual increase in my probing inward pressure. The mass was knobby and surprisingly hard. Encompassing its two- by four-inch bulk within my fingertips, I could move it very slightly from side to side but not up or down. It lay precisely where the stomach should have been, seeming to have pushed that organ out of its accustomed place, or perhaps actually to be enclosed within it. It took but a moment for me to recognize that reality had appeared with a crash—I had no idea what I was feeling in that little belly.

I was crestfallen. Clearly, I would be deprived of the grandeur of my anticipated dramatic moment, during which enlightenment was to have shone forth from me onto the small group awaiting my decisive pronouncement. The clinical wellspring had failed me. That sparkling divine source meant to nurture the lush groves of a surgeon's transcendent and self-evident superiority was dry. There would be no diagnostic victory that day.

I stood there for nearly another minute, reluctant to lift my hand from Clyde Jr.'s abdomen. Were I to look up at my expectant colleagues, I would then have to admit being no less puzzled than were any of the young pediatricians who had examined the child. What could possibly be the nature of a large, bulky structure within the abdomen of an infant that had not been present when the child was last examined only four weeks earlier? Buying time by pretending to continue my manual examination, I let my mind run rapidly through the drill physicians turn to when faced with the dilemma of trying to categorize a seemingly undiagnosable mass: is it congenital, neoplastic, traumatic, or inflammatory?

The likelihood of a congenital, or inborn, origin seemed virtually nil in light of the lump's previous absence; there is no neoplasm, or tumor, that might have grown so rapidly; the parents had denied trauma when questioned by the pediatricians, and there was no evidence of it on the child's body. An inflammatory cause—infectious, actually—seemed the least unlikely possibility, and might explain the temperature of 101° and the moderate elevation in white blood count reported by the lab. But the presence of infection would mean that the mass was most probably an abscess—a walled-off collection of pus—and what strange set of circumstances might be the source of such a thing in a child this age? And yet another argument, too, could be made against the diagnosis of abscess: being essentially a large, deeply seated boil and therefore tender to the touch, an abscess is usually painful when pressed upon. This baby had not reacted when I pushed against the mass. Just to be sure—and also to stall a bit longer—I exerted pressure on the distended little belly once more. Again, the child gave no indication of discomfort.

Finally, I could no longer justify further delay. I straightened up and, without saying a word, stepped outside the examining cubicle to speak with the young parents.

Nona, the mother, looked no more than a high schooler, and Clyde Sr., though in his mid-twenties, seemed not much older. My first impression was of a dulled blankness about both of them that I instantly knew would make effective communication difficult. It was as though they heard my brief greeting through a dense baffle that would obscure the meaning of my questions. Within a few moments, it became clear that they seemed not to understand why they were being quizzed at all, much less by one doctor after another.

Only the rail-thin Clyde Sr. spoke, while Nona just stared at me vacantly. He was tall and ungainly, his skinniness made skinnier by ill-fitting overalls and a loose T-shirt. Nevertheless, he was not without a certain lackluster handsomeness. His black hair was buzz-cut as if he were a new recruit to the Marines, and he did in fact slowly rotate a soiled olive-drab fatigue cap in his callused hands as he stood there, vaguely contemplating a spot located somewhere in the middle of my chest as he spoke. Standing so close to him that their sides touched, the slightly built Nona looked more a waif than a wife. Her uncombed wavy hair was a dirty blond color. Slouching posture accentuated the awkward bulging of her lower abdomen, a reminder of her recent pregnancy that even her loose, flowered pinafore could not hide. She might have been pretty had her face not been so utterly lifeless.

Neither Nona nor Clyde Sr. betrayed an iota of emotion. If they were worried about their child, their faces were too expressionless to reveal it.

Clyde Sr.'s answers came slowly and for the most part in monosyllables, doubtless from long habit. His responses were as spare as his body, and were delivered with the unmistakable twang of his Maine origins. All of these details come back to me along with that entire disconcerting sense of being thwarted at every turn, as I leaf through the pages of the baby's chart almost four decades later. Within the limits of what today feels like complete recall but must be only a reasonable approximation, this is what we said to each other:

"Before the diarrhea began, did you notice anything unusual about the baby in the past few weeks?"

"Nope."

"Has he had an elevated temperature, or seemed hot at any time?"

"Nope."

"Is it possible that he might have fallen from something, or been injured in any way?"

"Doubt it—mebbe when we wasn't lookin'."

"But you would have noticed something, or someone in the family would have told you."

"'Spect so, but they didn't. So I guess not. Ain't that right, Nona?"

She nodded.

"Has the baby seemed sick in any way?"

"Like we told them other doctors—Nope."

"If you should think of anything later that you've forgotten, you'll let us know, won't you?"

"Yup. Sure will."

The Greenes appeared to be insulated from the life around them. They stood there side by side, in a fog of opaque incomprehension that could not be fully explained by invoking mere Yankee taciturnity. Whether it was a mutuality of borderline intelligence or a chronicity of hopelessness—or both—I could not tell, but trying to get information out of these two was like squeezing blood out of the proverbial turnip.

In reading the report made by the social worker after her interview of Nona a few days later, I would learn more about her. The eldest of ten children born to farmers in rural Maine, she had left school in the eighth grade because, in her words, she "couldn't catch on." From then until her marriage to Clyde Sr. when she was three months pregnant, she passed the time by helping her mother with the other kids and picking berries and potatoes to earn money for the household.

Nona's relationship with her baby reflected her own immature uncertainty:

Mrs. Greene is a bland, apparently intellectually limited young woman who is somewhat passively dependent. I had the impression that she finds the hospital setting rather overwhelming . . . [She] presented herself as confused around how to manage a baby. She lacks the confidence to use her judgment . . . She has no friends with infants and is thus unable to get any suggestions or clues from them . . . During the day Mrs. Greene occasionally cuddles Clyde but usually he sleeps while she looks at TV or is reading pulp literature. It was learned that she felt confused about how to bathe Clyde; just when to hold or burp him; and is fearful of hurting him due to his small size . . . [I]t is difficult for the mother to be very spontaneous with him.

All of these statements were consistent with my impression of Nona that morning, and were of a piece with every contact she and I would have during Clyde Jr.'s week in the hospital.

When I went back into the examining room, a nurse was wrapping the baby in preparation for his transportation to the x-ray suite. Now chastened and stripped of my air of self-importance, I spoke briefly— and with new humility—to the chief pediatric resident, and then went back to the OR to begin my second case of the day. As much as he wanted to learn the diagnosis, my pediatric counterpart seemed relieved that it would not be coming from *me*.

On emerging from the OR two hours later, I was handed a message from one of the residents on the radiology service. He wanted me to come downstairs to his department as soon as I could, to look at the child's films with him. The secretary taking the message had written that his concluding words were, "Tell him he won't believe this."

The films were up on the lighted screen when I arrived in the x-ray suite a few minutes later. The radiology resident had been showing them to colleagues, students, technicians—virtually anyone who passed by. As I walked into the large open viewing area, I could see the focus of his astonishment from fifty feet away. Filling almost the entire stomach of the baby was a large, dense object that looked exactly like a lobulated stone. Alongside the first film of the abdomen were two other pictures, taken after Clyde Jr. had been fed a bit of soda water. The gas released from the drink outlined the foreign body with striking clarity. It matched precisely the mass that had been felt on physical examination, but its appearance did not help to answer the question of what it might possibly be.

The radiologist had been delaying the dictation of his final report, hoping that I would be able to provide further information that might clarify the nature of his finding. He was disappointed to hear that I could tell him nothing beyond what the pediatricians had already reported. The following are the first sentences he now spoke into the recording microphone as I stood beside him, still trying to puzzle the thing out. I have transcribed them from his report as it appears in Clyde Jr.'s chart:

> A large 5 by 5 by 9 centimeter mass forming a concretion [a solid stonelike mass] which fills the stomach is demonstrated in the left upper quadrant. Additional films were obtained with a carbinated [*sic*] liquid which forms a clearer outline of the solid boundaries of this foreign body. This bezoar appears to terminate at the area of the pylorus [the narrow exit channel of the stomach].

Bezoar—an oddity mentioned in passing one day in class during the second year of medical school, but not something one expected to encounter in the realities of clinical life. The fourteen-hundred-page pathology textbook I used during my residency devoted a single paragraph to bezoars, and even that bit was printed in small type to denote rarity. But the bezoar's very peculiarity always causes medical students to remember it, regardless of its seeming insignificance in the enormous catalog of abnormalities they must carry in their heads. When I later wrote my surgical consultation note in the baby's chart, it began with the words "Wonder of wonders!"

A bezoar is a foreign body that forms in the stomach when indigestible swallowed material conglomerates and cannot be passed out through the pylorus and on into the small intestine. In the Middle Ages and for centuries afterward, bezoars retrieved from the stomachs of animals were thought to have magical properties, especially against poisons. The notion lives on today in the form of belief in amulets and lucky stones and even rabbits' feet. When found in human beings, these concretions are most commonly composed of hair that a troubled young person has pulled from his own head and then ingested. This variety is called a trichobezoar to distinguish it from those made up of fruit and vegetable fibers, known as phytobezoars (from the Greek words for "hair" and "plant," respectively). Concretions of shellac and similar materials have also been found in the stomachs of disturbed patients.

All of this was well known to each of us who reviewed the baby's films, in spite of our absolute innocence of any previous experience with it. What was not known—and could not even be imagined—was the origin of this incomprehensible clump that was obstructing the stomach of our little patient.

I went down to the emergency room to quiz the Greenes again, but they had hurriedly taken off for home as soon as the baby was transported to the x-ray department. When I phoned them, Nona answered and informed me that they had left because no one had specifically told them to stay, "and anyways, Clyde had to get back to the lumberyard." I asked that they return, and then phoned the OR to schedule the operation the child would so obviously need.

About twenty minutes later, Nona came in without Clyde but accompanied by her sister-in-law, a sullen, rawboned woman incongruously named Merry ("Merry," though a *pseudo*nym, is also a *syno*nym for this ill-humored woman's real name). Though perhaps only about ten years older than the baby's mother, Merry looked and acted more like an overbearing stepmother than she did a supportive sister-in-law. Each question I asked of Nona was answered abruptly by the older woman until, growing annoyed and impatient, I insisted that the baby's mother speak for herself. The grudgingly accepted switch in respondents made no difference, except that it added to the enmity of the sister-in-law, who was already suspicious of my motives in asking so many questions, "when all you have to do is take care of the kid. If he needs an operation, well then go ahead, why don'tcha?"

Both Nona and Merry denied the possibility of Clyde Jr.'s having been fed any of a variety of substances I named that might have formed a bezoar. Though they claimed to be certain, I could not help but feel uneasy. It was not their motives that I mistrusted, but their competence. In spite of her stolid appearance of disdainful self-assurance, Merry seemed not much more capable than her chronically dazed sister-in-law.

Still unenlightened, I made the only decision I could: to take our little charge off to the OR without further delay. By then, his story had attracted the attention of a number of members of the medical staff, who had heard about it not only from the pediatricians but also via the senior attending surgeon from whom I had vainly sought further suggestions. He had, in fact, turned to another of those stratagems used by physicians in tight situations, as the pediatricians had done earlier when they obtained the X ray and a consultation. On hearing the details of the puzzle confronting us, he had invoked the time-honored maxim to which members of our craft resort when faced with the impossibility of a diagnosis: "When evaluating an abdominal problem in the emergency room," he had intoned as though reciting scripture, "a surgeon can get along perfectly well without a plan, and even without a diagnosis, providing he can make three decisions correctly: One, should this patient be admitted? Two, should this patient have an operation? Three, what incision should I make? If he gets those things right, he'll find out everything he needs to know once he has the belly open." As of that day, I had already during the four previous years of my training had many opportunities to test the indisputable logic of this kind of thinking, and had not yet known it to fail. Armed with the professor's go-ahead and reassured by the fact of his being as stymied as the rest of us, I changed into a clean pair of greens and began the ritual of scrubbing, surrounded on each side by young men who were, like me, each in a high state of anticipation.

All sorts of conjectures were being floated throughout the hospital about what we would find in Clyde Jr.'s stomach and where it might turn out to have come from. The guesses ranged in usefulness from the sober and thoughtful to the wild and wiseacre. My own diagnosis was based on my impression of the Greenes. Despite their denials, I was convinced that they had fed the child some esoteric Maine backwoods nostrum, intended in some mystical way to build up his scrawny preemie's body. Being quite obviously odd, unworldly, and not very bright, they seemed a good bet to be superstitious too. I expected to find a solid glob of occult New England witches' brew coagulated in the baby's stomach.

After Clyde Jr. was transferred onto the operating table, the surgical intern injected a bit of local anesthetic into the skin over an ankle vein and made a short incision allowing the insertion of a length of poly-ethylene tubing for the infusion of fluids. Until then, hydration had been accomplished through a forearm intravenous needle placed in the emergency room by the pediatricians.

Because he was concerned that his patient might vomit during in-duction, the anesthesiologist slid a tiny breathing tube into the baby's windpipe while he was still awake. Not unexpectedly, Clyde Jr. reacted to this intrusion of his airway by coughing violently, resulting in the forceful expulsion of the tube. When a second attempt failed in the same way, the anesthesiologist stopped trying and reached for the ether can. Ether was being used almost exclusively for the anesthe-sia of infants at Yale–New Haven at the time, and the struggling little patient was now induced by dripping the volatile liquid from the small container onto a gauze mask positioned snugly over his face. When Clyde Jr. seemed deep enough into etherized sleep, the breathing tube was inserted and securely taped into place. The baby's protuberant ab-domen was swabbed with antiseptic solution by the medical student, and pediatric towels and drapes were applied. They were positioned in such a way that a small aperture exposed the upper abdomen.

As we took our places at the operating table, one of the junior resi-dents delivered himself of the weighty opinion that he was sure we would find a Maine potato in our patient's stomach, picked specially for him by his slow-witted mother. "And you can bet it'll be half-baked," he added. The intern, a New Englander himself, chimed in that it had to be a piece of scrimshaw, carved for his firstborn by Clyde Sr. as a good luck charm. Hearing all of this, and still annoyed with himself for his inability to intubate the baby while awake, the anesthesiologist mumbled something obscene and told us to get on with the operation.

I made a short transverse incision in the skin over the mass, and car-ried it through the sparse fatty layer beneath. After cutting through the underlying muscle, I opened the inner envelope of fibrous tis-sue—the peritoneum—and entered the abdominal cavity. There ex-posed in front of me lay the bulging stomach, so packed with its mysterious content that a lumpy protrusion in its center was pushing up toward me, as though pointing out where I should place the cutting edge of my scalpel.

The human stomach is held only loosely by its broad attachments of fat-streaked pliant folds of tissue called the omentum. Because the omentum of a seven-pound infant is flimsy and flexible, it was a simple matter to displace the stomach forward toward me and bring it out to the surface through the widely spread opening I had made in the layers of the abdominal wall.

The puzzle was about to be solved. I asked the assembled team and our onlookers for any last-second guesses before beginning to make my way through the fleshy wall of the stomach. Eager to know the answer at last, no one seemed keen to waste any further time coming up with abstruse diagnoses or attempts at humor. The room was silent.

By "make my way," I mean exactly what those three words imply. The gastric (from the Greek *gaster*, meaning "the belly," but understood to refer exclusively to the stomach) wall has three separate and rather thick circumferential coats, two of which are composed of several distinct layers fed by a very abundant blood supply, as befits an organ that has a lot of work to do. To "make my way" through these layers it was necessary to clamp and then tie the small vessels as I encountered them, each with a meticulously applied ligature of fine silk. By the time I reached the innermost layer of the organ's lining (called the mucosa or mucous membrane), I could almost literally feel the hot breath of several of the huddled group of pediatric residents on the back of my neck.

At last, I cut through the final bit—and there lay the prize. In the words of the operative note I dictated immediately after completing the surgery: "The bezoar revealed itself to be a large irregular white structure which resembled nothing so much as a chewed-up lump of wax." Rather than unnecessarily enlarge the gastric incision in order to remove the mass, I simply broke up the amorphous thing with a clamp into a large number of fragments, which could then be scooped up with a spoonlike instrument and laid out onto the surgical drape. Lying there on the green cloth, they resembled clumps of candle wax. As a child, I would sometimes amuse myself by biting off the end of one of my grandmother's Sabbath candles and grinding it up between my teeth, finally spitting the pieces into the sink. The bits I was now picking up off the drape and holding in my gloved hand looked and felt exactly like those long-forgotten fragments of white tallow.

Finally, I knew what was in the stomach. But I still had no idea of how it had gotten there, and neither did anyone else in that room. In the gaggle of voices that now filled the air, I heard not a word that might enlighten me. Once again, the moment that I had expected to be definitive was instead frustrating. I felt stymied, especially since I was certain that further questioning of the obtusely unhelpful Greenes would only leave me again dissatisfied.

But before I could return to face the blank expressions of the parents and the overt antagonism of Aunt Merry, there was work still to be done in the operating room. When a patient, particularly a young child, accumulates a substance of any nature in its stomach, the possibility must be considered that some kind of obstruction is preventing normal passage into the intestine. With Clyde Jr., the abnormality uppermost in the minds of all of us was the condition known as pyloric stenosis, whose characteristic subject is a firstborn boy approximately two to three weeks old. This is a congenital disease in which the circle of muscle in the wall of the pylorus is greatly thickened (the medical word is *hypertrophied*), to such a degree that little or no material can pass through the narrowed channel and on into the intestine.

With the stomach lying open there before me, it was not difficult to convince myself that there was no evidence of pyloric stenosis, nor did any type of bandlike congenital abnormality exist that might impede the egress of gastric contents. Not only was the pylorus not thickened but I could easily pass my fifth finger through its wide-open channel and into the duodenum, the uppermost segment of the intestine. I then slid a wide rubber catheter all the way around to the far end of the duodenum to prove the absence of any obstruction further down. The remainder of the intestinal tract appeared normal in every way. After washing each last bit of waxy bezoar out of the stomach, I sutured up the opening I had made in its wall, and then closed the abdominal incision in layers of fine silk stitches.

As expected, further questioning of the three Greenes got me nowhere. The baby did well postoperatively and was discharged a week after the surgery. There was no recurrence of the problem.

Late on the afternoon before Clyde Jr.'s discharge, I wandered into the room he shared with three other little kids and set myself down on a small chair facing his mother. I had come upon her sitting alone there, her lusterless eyes fixed on a page of one of those tattered, long-outdated magazines that are such an integral part of the furnishings of every hospital in America. Clyde Jr. was peacefully asleep. Having unexpectedly found her, I seized on this last opportunity for getting to the bottom of what had by then become the great riddle of the pediatric and surgery departments. If I could solve it, I would, at the last moment, achieve at least some modicum of the victory over my "cognitive" colleagues that had eluded me when I examined the child in the emergency room.

Although I expected nothing to come of the attempt, I began by asking Nona to tell me how she prepared the formula for her baby. Perhaps I thought she might divulge the name of some ingredient not meant to be part of the feeding, but I don't specifically recall that to be my motive. Very likely, I was just looking for stones—literally and figuratively—that might not have been previously turned over. Although she had been quizzed repeatedly about every possibility of an abnormal substance entering Clyde Jr.'s mouth, it had not occurred to any of us that we should question his routine intake. Was it possible that this clueless girl was somehow doing something peculiar in her formula preparation, knowledge of which might lead to the solution of our continuing conundrum?

"Well, I ain't been usin' the formula, and that's 'cause Merry tol' me not to. She says a baby needs real milk and that's what I been givin' him." Her voice trailing off as though in uncertainty, she added, "'Cause that's what she said is right, that's why I do like that." She was almost inaudible at the last few words.

I remembered a comment in the social worker's report, in a paragraph headed "Mrs. Greene's Handling of Clyde." Immediately following the statement about Nona's confusion in managing her infant were a few thoughts that might provide the key to the bezoar's origin. The first sentences of the pertinent paragraph appear in the chart as follows:

> *Mrs. Greene's Handling of Clyde* Mrs. Greene presented herself as confused around how to manage a baby. She lacks the confidence to use her judgement in the face of her sister-in-law's suggestions. Those suggestions have on occasion been in contradiction to recommendations from doctors. When such occasions occur Mrs. Greene usually takes her sister-in-law's advice. Although she expressed no resentment of her sister-in-law's interference it was my impression that Mrs. Greene is beginning to tire of this help from her relative. She has no friends with infants and is thus unable to get any suggestions or clues from them. Apparently her mother's handling of her siblings varies sharply also with the handling doctors have suggested.

All at once I felt like a detective on the trail of a hot clue. In those few sentences might be the explanation for Nona's disregard of the feeding instructions she had been given on bringing her newborn home. In answer to my next question, she took me through her routine preparation of the whole milk she had been feeding her baby: "Well, after I get the water to boil in the pot, I put the container of milk right in there so's it gets warm. That's how my ma did it too, and I always did it for the little kids back home, 'cept we don't get milk in no containers in Maine, so I have to be careful to do it just right."

The year was 1961—cardboard dairy containers were not yet in universal use. In rural areas of New England, all milk was still being delivered in glass bottles. I asked Nona whether she had been heating containered milk in boiling water since bringing her baby home from the hospital. The answer came in a single laconic word: "Yup." I excused myself and left the room to find the head nurse.

Within thirty minutes Nona had been instructed—reinstructed, actually—in formula preparation and the absolute necessity that she not feed her baby whole milk, and in any event never to heat any form of food in a cardboard container. I could at least hope that telling Nona my explanation for the origin of the bezoar would convince her that the time had come to assert some independence from the overbearing Merry and the example of her own mother.

Of course, I will never know for sure whether I really did find the correct solution to the puzzle, but it made sense to me then and it makes sense to me now, as it did to the pediatricians when I told them about Nona's practices. As we reconstructed it, minute globules of the wax lining the inside of the container were being melted off by the heat of the boiling water and passing directly into the milk. Once the collection of indigestible wax in the infant's little stomach had become just large enough to cause even a minor degree of partial obstruction of the pylorus, buildup became rapid. In time blocking all egress, the whole mass had come to be shaped like an undersized Maine potato.

CHAPTER TWO

THE STOMACH:

SOUL, SPIRIT,

AND CENTRALITY

T HOUGH we pay them no mind, the flowings of life can be sensed within us. Deliberate concentration or specific circumstances may be required to bring them to overt attention, but the intermittent gurgles or quickening—and sometimes even the muffled pulsing beat of inner currents—are familiar to our deepest unthinking perception. So accustomed are we to an intangible awareness of the regular stream of messages rising up from within our bodies that the most subtle alteration in their accustomed character comes immediately to consciousness, telling us that a physical change has somewhere taken place. Even the meaning of the change can be understood: whether cause for concern or just another of the waxing and waning fluxes of a normal day's ceaseless activity in the cavernous abdominal depths or the ribbed enclosure of the chest; whether the something new is warning of a matter amiss or bears only the familiar resonance of mere adjustment in the service of a transitory visceral necessity.

Some communiqués from within are of an urgent sort. The determined trumpetings of nausea, pain, or hunger require no fine discrimination to interpret. Whether pleas or orders, they demand response. Our bodies count on their unmistakable clarity to signal that something must be done, and soon. These are overtly discernible calls of distress, not to be ignored.

The variety of messages generated from our depths has been the subject of conjecture since our species or perhaps its most advanced forebears first appeared. When the Greek physician Galen wrote nearly two millennia ago, "In the body of an animal, there is nothing inert, nothing motionless," he was only telling his readers what every sentient beast already knew: There is a lot going on down there, and it seems independent of our will or control. If we pay attention, we can pick up signals that are clues to life itself.

It was the seeming independence of our inner dynamism that must have caused the peoples of ancient times to assume that the capacious cavities of their bellies and chests were the site of activities not only physical but mystical as well. In early history, and in more recent folk societies too, the entire surrounding universe has been thought to be awash with magical determinants of common phenomena. There was an assumption of spiritual forces abroad in every forest and glen, and a sky full of temperamental gods who observe each man's actions and manipulate his destiny. How else to explain the vagaries of fortune, health, weather, famines, and floods?

It is only natural that the churning of viscera should have been subject to the same kind of interpretation. If the actions of sprites, spirits, and gods functioning outside of him affect a man's fate, perhaps there are factors in his organs, too, that influence the type of person he is and his behavior. Tens of centuries before people looked to genes as determinants of all manner of personal characteristics, they looked to their guts. But in those days little was known of the mysterious inner forces they sought to understand. Fanciful theories abounded over just what it is that goes on beneath the layers of skin, fat, and fiber hiding a man's deepest parts from his own direct scrutiny. The ancient Egyptians, for example, believed that an independent life was being lived by some of the larger, identifiable structures inside them—such as the heart, the uterus, the stomach, and some of the major blood vessels. These and others were said to wander freely about the chest and abdomen when the inclination struck them, like independent creatures answering only to their own changing moods or whims. The Babylonians, at a loss to identify the whys and wherefores of mental processes, sought explanations in the activities of certain of their viscera, from which they convinced themselves that thoughts originate. To those who rested by the waters of Babylon, the heart was the seat of the intellect, the uterus of compassion, and the liver of mood. Though the captive Hebrew psalmist may have admonished himself, "If I forget thee, O Jerusalem, let my right hand forget her cunning," the ultimate source of that cunning was certified by the locals to reside in the stomach.

It was not uncommon in those distant days that a man's belly was laid open by beast or battle, or the inside of his chest exposed by an attacker's slashing weapon. A bold and inquisitive onlooker might then briefly observe the compressive undulations of a few yards of coiled intestine or watch a vanquished heart as it beat until its regularity broke up into an uncoordinated maelstrom of irregular wrigglings, finally becoming stilled forever. When animals were killed for food and their innards cut or torn out, it could be verified that their body cavities were packed tightly with viscera much like those of the men who were gutting them. Knowledge of human anatomy gradually expanded in this way, by reasoning from butchered to butcher. No one ever saw a spleen or a uterus actually move, but who could know what those compact units of fleshy independence might be doing when unobserved in their clandestine precincts?

Perhaps most remarkable to primitive or ancient observers was the variation between one organ and another. The purple-gray, spongy spleen was so different in appearance and texture from the serpentine, squishy bowel or the rubbery, yellow-brown solidity of the liver. Each viscus seemed an individual, very like a distinctive person with distinctive characteristics. For these reasons, the various structures were thought to impart distinctive personality characteristics as well to those who harbored them in the protected confines of the two huge body cavities.

As early societies developed institutions and in time created systems of law and commerce, religious beliefs became more complex, but no less imaginative. Explanations of natural phenomena remained embroiled in mysticism and fancy. Increasingly, the sources of variations in human behavior were sought in the differing characteristics of the organs and fluids of the trunk and also in the gelatinous convolutions of the brain. Individual societies found their own notions of how to interpret what they saw and felt, not only about the qualities of character imparted by those organs but by their usefulness in human functioning as well. How, for example, could the presence of the spleen be accounted for? When the slit-open belly of a slaughtered animal—or a slaughtered man—was inspected, the spleen was found tucked up almost out of sight, high under the left leaf of the diaphragm. What was it doing there? Being so close to the stomach, it was thought by the Greeks to have some effect on the newly swallowed food, but what could that effect be? The spleen's dark somberness gave it an aura of funereal solemnity amidst the more lively hues of the structures nearby—perhaps it was the seat of melancholy.

Or the liver, forcefully pushing its huge tan bulk downward against its lesser neighbors and pressing into the diaphragm and lung above, as befits its seeming suzerainty of the belly's upper reaches—the uniqueness of its massive authority was unquestioned. Recognized by most early observers to be the place where all blood is received, it was thought by many to be the site of its manufacture. Blood being so obviously the focus of life, the liver's predominance was such that priests and magicians would search its lobular structure for signs and portents when an animal was sacrificed or slaughtered for food. There is an aura of boldness surrounding the liver's assertion of its hegemony. Surely, thought those who contemplated its regal expansiveness, the abundant clear yellow fluid that comes forth from its depths must transmit that boldness to the entire man, imparting to him certain qualities that reflect the temperament of the liver itself.

The origins of such schemata are lost in the misted obscurities of earliest civilizations, but vestiges of them can be found in the discovered traditions of the Fertile Crescent and later in Egypt. Egyptian physicians traveled to Arabia, Persia, and Greece, their medical

philosophies becoming intermingled with those of the newer civilizations. An example of their influence as teachers may be found in the
heritage of Hippocrates himself, whose physician grandfather—also
named Hippocrates—was the pupil of an Egyptian. In such ways, the
old knowledge was preserved, handed down as family tradition from
father to son as it was from society to society. Like the theoretical
power of the liver's yellow bile, the notion of formative fluids called
humors traveling throughout the body was brought to the Ionian
peninsula, as was so much of the lore of preceding cultures in another
way too, via the maritime travels of Greek traders and the migration of
small societies. All primitive medicine being based on magic and religious belief, the Greeks were the recipients of a hodgepodge of formulations, not only concerning the activities of the internal organs
but about their anatomy as well.

It was characteristic of these times that metaphysical constructs
were decisive, even when they defied the reality of what could be seen.
When observed phenomena did not match the conceptions of the
priests, hypothetical structures, functions, and fluids were invented to
fit into accepted structures of belief. Humankind will never be free of
such patterns of preconceived thought. Traces—and sometimes far
more than traces—of similar methods of justification are still discoverable in many of the nonstandard healing practices of today. They
have been at the foundation of entire philosophies of sickness and
cure.

Like the civilizations before them, the Greeks lived in thrall to mystical concepts of disease and health for hundreds of years before the
golden age of their greatest philosophical and literary accomplishments in the fifth and fourth centuries B.C.E. Though modified somewhat by their own unique additions, their medicine's supernatural
foundation was essentially of a piece with the accumulated lore of
their predecessors. They sought healing in temples dedicated to the
powers of the god Aesculapius and his children, among whom
his daughters Hygeia and Panacea were the most prominent. The
sonorous voices of the priests echoed through the open spaces within
those dedicated shrines, where sacred snakes, visionary dreams, and
votive offerings were the keys to recovery.

When in the fifth century B.C.E. Greek physicians began to create what has come to be called the medicine of Hippocrates—a method of healing based on direct observation and the exclusion of the super-natural—they nevertheless remained heir to formulations whose origins are discoverable in the very theurgy they were determined to expunge. As accurate as were their observations of natural phenomena, these later Greeks not infrequently explained what they saw by attributing fanciful characteristics to body parts and fluids, just as had the superstitious healers before them. Paramount in their ideas of physiology was the principle that the action of the fluids known as humors determines not only one's state of health, but even one's temperament. As was true of the vestiges of their continuing belief in the specific personalities of the organs themselves, they adapted these notions from similar beliefs of earlier civilizations and even from certain traits they continued to attribute to the organs in which the fluids were said to originate.

There are lessons in contemplating the Greek absorption of non-rational ideas into a system of medicine that historians are fond of hailing as rational. No matter the insistence of philosophers that objectivity and reason can replace emotionalism and tradition; no matter the homage we pay to the scientific method, new paradigms of detached fact-gathering, and a resolute rejection of a long tradition of magical thinking—no matter any of these determined seekings for a civilization guided by reason, there are inherent currents within the mind of *Homo sapiens* that will not be denied. Not only do cultures build their present on the past, but they retain certain fundamental elements universal to our species. Among them is the inborn sense of forces beyond our ken, forces that may be welcomed as a child welcomes a father's nurturing or feared as a child fears a father's punishing and sometimes capricious nature. What has come before in a society is borne by powerful psychological currents into the present. As individuals, we are made of the urgencies of today and the memories of yesterday; as societies, we never relinquish the formative shapings of history and the perceptions and yearnings within the psyche of each individual, even when we seem to be unaware of them—at least in the sense that they do not rise to consciousness. Only in mythology does a phoenix fly free of its incinerated past and its fleshly being. In real life, the past and our basic nature are always with us, not as dead ashes but in the form of motivating currents flowing into the structure of our daily lives.

Within every modern person are irrational forces—whatever the depth of their submersion—that frustrate our puny attempts to shake off their unacknowledged power over us. Even the Greeks, those stalwarts of golden reason, absorbed and reconfigured their full share of magical thinking, weaving it seamlessly into their medicine. When the eminent Swiss historian of the mid-twentieth century, Erwin Ackerknecht, referred to the writings of the Hippocratic physicians as "medicine's Declaration of Independence" from religion and superstition, he was not completely correct; he gave the mind of man more credit than it deserves. Superstition, tradition, wishful thinking, and baseless hypothesis have not only always lived alongside science but have been interlarded with it to a much greater degree than even thoughtful critics are often willing to concede. In denying the obvious, they too are indulging themselves in a kind of wishful thinking.

So commanding and durable would the belief in the physiological influence of the designated humors become that it outlasted every European empire from the Greek to the Napoleonic. Not until after the middle of the nineteenth century was scientific medicine sufficiently authoritative to replace it as the foundation of therapeutic methodology for all Western-trained physicians. In various guises and in the closely related form of hypothetical types of energy, the balance of fluids or forces remains today the guiding principle of certain nonscientific healing practices.

Modern biomedical science, too, sometimes flirts with similar slumbering archaisms. In contemplating such twentieth-century discoveries as hormones, signaling molecules, and that bulwark of resistance to disease that they have provocatively named humoral immunity, the apostles of modernity pay homage of a sort—even if only in terminology—to the old tradition. In their commitment to the principle of homeostasis, or internal equilibrium, they positively embrace it. In all of these ways, the humoral concept of the Greeks is still with us, muted and disguised but always lurking in the shadowed background of our minds.

ALTHOUGH the theory of humors has been applied during antiquity—and since—in complex and sometimes contradictory ways, it can be resolved into a few rather simple principles.

According to the magisterial physician Galen, who codified the theory for posterity in the second century C.E., the body has within it four liquids, or humors, each imparting specific characteristics that are not only physical but mental as well. The four were said to exist together in a coordinated balance that maintains health and emotional stability. But should one or another of them become altered in quantity or quality, the result is disease or changes in personality. The four are blood, yellow bile, black bile, and phlegm.

The notion of the four humors is related to a doctrine developed in the fifth century B.C.E. by the Sicilian natural philosopher Empedocles. Empedocles taught that all matter is composed of one or more of four elements: fire, air, earth, and water, which he believed to be the "root of all things." These four were attracted to and repulsed by one another by means of the opposing forces of Love and Hate, the various combinations and separations resulting in the many forms of matter. The four elements were, in turn, believed to correspond to the four qualities of hot, dry, cold, and wet.

Blood was thought to come forth from the heart, and therefore to be wet and hot; yellow bile originates in the liver, and is dry and hot; black bile comes from the spleen and stomach, and is dry and cold; phlegm comes from the brain, and is wet and cold. The relationships of the humors to the various factors may be diagrammed as follows:

ELEMENT	QUALITY	HUMOR	CHARACTERISTICS	SOURCE
Fire	hot	blood	wet and hot	heart
Air	dry	yellow bile	dry and hot	liver
Earth	cold	black bile	dry and cold	spleen, stomach
Water	wet	phlegm	wet and cold	brain

In this system, each humor has its own effect on behavior and health. Blood quickens the spirit; yellow bile emboldens it; black bile makes it stolid and melancholy; and phlegm makes it sluggish. These formulations have survived in our language in the form of common adjectives derived from Greek or Latin origins. *Sanguine* (from the Latin *sanguis,* or "blood") means "lively," "ardent," or "optimistic"; *choleric* (from the Greek *chole,* or "bile") means "easily angered" or "irritated," while *bilious* (from the Latin *bilis,* or "bile" or "gall") means "ill-tempered" or "cross"; *melancholic* (from the Greek *melas,* or "black," and *chole*) means "gloomy" or "depressed"; *phlegmatic* (from the Greek *phlegma,* or "a fire" or "heat") means "dull" and "sluggish," but also "calm" and "imperturbable."

(An intriguing evolution has occurred in the significance of "spleen" and "splenic." Originally, an attack of spleen meant a period of melancholy, and a person so afflicted was sad or depressed—his black bile was overabundant. That meaning is now archaic. Over the centuries, "spleen" and "splenic" [as well as "splenetic," which is derived from them] have come to take on a different connotation, so that nowadays an attack of spleen is understood to be a fit of anger, and to vent one's spleen is to let the anger out and thus relieve emotional tension. The etymology of the term implies a recognition that internalized anger can cause psychiatric depression. It is avoided by letting the anger out.)

Every individual was believed to have his own distinct quantity of each humor; the proportions of the mixture determined baseline personality, since each person has his own unique balance of the four. Disease occurs when one's balance is upset. Even hour-by-hour mood is affected by small fluctuations in the equilibrium. Simple observation indicates that behavior may vary somewhat depending on the time of year, as well. The Greeks attributed this to seasonal elevations in one or another humor: blood increases in the spring (a young man's fancy lightly turns to thoughts of love), yellow bile in the summer (the frictions of a long, hot summer), black bile in the autumn (fall, the season of depression), and phlegm in the winter (obvious from the frequency of runny noses).

In developing the thesis that disease was due not to the intervention of gods but to imbalance in the humors, the followers of Hippocrates did, as Ackerknecht pointed out, assert a degree of independence from the supernatural. But like the systems that preceded theirs, the theory of humors came into being because the Greeks were not content to leave anything unexplained. Unlike modern science, whose greatest strength may be its willingness to confess any present ignorance, the ancients insisted that all-inclusive explanations must exist for every phenomenon. Such a perspective results in the filling in of gaps with inchoate hypothetical notions based on shaky evidence, inaccurate interpretation of observations, or sheer invention—a practice that has characterized every nonscientific system of healing up to the present time. For the Greeks, and for many of the healing philosophies of every era, this meant the substitution of the fanciful for the mystical—the replacement of magic by imagination. Although the humors were real, the properties attributed to them were not. An entire catalog of folk and traditional medicine could be listed here whose adherents have allowed themselves to fall prey to similarly fallacious reasoning.

If the gods did not influence humoral imbalance, what did? The Greek answer to this question developed from the scrupulous attention they paid to the analysis of their own experience and its relation to their observations of the world around them. Trauma, the phenomena of nature such as weather, climate, surroundings, inborn personal characteristics, life experiences—these were the kinds of things that could be seen to be related to changes in health. Since sickness was the result of disequilibrium, restoring health meant restoring the balance of humors. Cure was accordingly sought through dietary measures, rest, withdrawal to a salubrious climate, and other more vigorous means of returning to the natural baseline. Because a surfeit of blood was such a common component of various disease states, bleeding—whether by lancet or leech—was the most useful stratagem of treatment. The laxatives, enemas, emetics, and similar obnoxious remedies so well remembered by an older generation today also have their origin in the heroic purging and puking of earlier times, all in the name of ridding the body of its overabundances. Such relatively recent modalities as mustard plasters, cupping, and counterirritant liniments originated in millennia-old attempts to draw excess humors, especially blood, upward to the surface and away from the interior depths where they might do the most harm.

Reliance on the theory of humors to explain disease was largely the result of the ancient physician's inability to study the functions of the actual organs directly, as well as a lack of will to do so. Whether from fear or awe, dissection of the human body was not practiced by the Greeks, except in a few unusual circumstances. Whatever knowledge of anatomy existed came from occasional studies of animals. Even these, unless in the hands of rare and remarkable individuals like Aristotle and later Galen, seem not to have been done according to any systematic scheme by which useful information could be gathered and collated. It might be thought that the embalming practices of the Egyptians should have provided the opportunity to learn more, but these procedures were carried out by the equivalent of technicians, who had no training or interest in adding to the fund of knowledge, such as it was. Explaining sickness and health by attributing hypothetical characteristics to certain fluids not only provided an all-inclusive theory but rendered unnecessary and even superfluous the careful study of organs.

Here again can be found a universal characteristic of non-Western systems of healing. Scientific medicine is the only tradition in which knowledge of the body's actual structure and functioning is acknowledged not only as the basis of understanding disease but also as something unattainable without dissection of the dead and study of the living, whether at surgery or by means of various biochemical or imaging techniques. Since other systems do not rely on directing therapy at specific well-identified abnormalities within individual organs, detailed knowledge is superfluous and useless to them. Like humoral medicine, such schemes depend for their efficacy on generalized readjustments of entire conditions of constitutional abnormality. The attitude of non-Western healers toward the specifics of anatomy and physiology is perhaps best summed up in a brief statement made to me by a Chinese colleague a few years ago, while I was visiting him at a medical school in Hunan province. Trying to explain the complexities of his country's five-thousand-year-old traditional medicine, this Western-trained surgeon found a way to clarify the subject: "When they talk about the liver or the thyroid, for instance," he said of China's traditional healers, "they don't mean the organ itself. What they are referring to is the *idea* of the organ. That's a very different thing. For that, anatomy is not needed."

The tradition of accurate knowledge can be said to have begun with Aristotle, whose descriptions of animal dissection and vivisection are the oldest we have. Ironically, Aristotle, who was a young man when Hippocrates died in approximately 370 B.C.E., was writing these descriptions precisely at the same time that the humor-based medicine of the Hippocratic physicians was spreading rapidly through the Greek territories. But his studies did not encourage others to emulate him. He remained a singular source of thought, but not an exemplar who would inspire others to continue his experimental ways. Even certain studies of human anatomy done about a century later by two trail-blazing and uniquely courageous Alexandrian physicians, Herophilus and Erasistratus, had no effect on medical theory, because they were suppressed and not rediscovered until much later.

But there was one structure whose usefulness and functioning seemed self-evident, even to the less sophisticated societies preceding the Greeks. It was perfectly clear that the pouchlike receptacle that is the stomach plays a vital role in determining at least the physical makeup of an individual. When Anthelme Brillat-Savarin wrote in 1825, "Tell me what you eat and I will tell you what you are," that urbane French gastronome knew that his *bon mot* went well beyond mere social context. Even as he was stating it, his aphorism was being taken quite literally by the medical profession of his day. Some of the physicians of the time went even further. It was the contention of the eminent London surgical teacher John Abernethy, for example, that there exists what he called a "reciprocal sympathy" between the digestive organs and the nervous system. His widely read 1809 book, *Surgical Observations,* provides plenty of dietary advice, which is in keeping with its thesis that problems with digestion produce generalized nervous disorders that in turn result in the localized diseases of one or another organ that physicians are called upon to treat.

Since prehistory, the evidence for Brillat-Savarin's aphorism had been there for all to see: A tempting delicacy is placed into the mouth, pleasurably savored, chewed, and then swallowed with enjoyment, usually in the society of others. Some hours or a day later, now in seclusion, its residuum is extruded from a concealed nether opening as a loathsome, foul-smelling mass of compacted brown muck, all of its tasty goodness having been extracted for conversion into the substance and energy that sustain the body. As so trenchantly put by the seventeenth-century English divine Edward Reynoldes, "We love our food when it is meate, we loathe it when it is excrement. When it goes into us we desire it, when it passeth through we despise it."

Should one ignore the importuning of the gut by not eating, the certain consequences will be dehydration, weight loss, wasting, and finally death, often preceded by the advent of some specific disease against which its malnourished victim is too debilitated to mount a successful counterattack. For thousands of years before Brillat-Savarin's birth, it had always been a matter of simple common sense: Whatever may be the contribution of forest elves or celestial supernature, we are what we eat. When we decrease our intake of food, our body size decreases too. If we put nothing into our stomachs, we will shrivel up and die.

From man's earliest and even fragmentary knowledge of his innards, he has been aware that the stomach is central to this sequence of intake and processing. Galen went so far as to attribute crucial significance not only to the stomach's function but even to its location, saying of the organ that it is the "central storehouse established in the middle of the animal for the benefit of all the parts." As he saw things, its centrality was magnified by its job. "This storehouse, a work of divine, not human, art, receives all the nutriment and subjects the food to its first elaboration, without which it would be useless and of no benefit to the animal. For just as workmen skilled in preparing wheat cleanse it of any earth, stones, or foreign seeds mixed with it that would be harmful to the body, so the faculty of the stomach thrusts downward [for elimination via the bowel] anything of that sort, but makes all the rest of the material, that is naturally good, still better and distributes it to the veins."

It was Galen's belief that the food was acted upon in the stomach by a process he named coction (alternatively called concoction), a term essentially interchangeable with "cooking." By this means, which utilizes a combination of grinding and the stomach's heat, food is converted into a thick liquid called chyle. According to this scheme, the stomach then attracts into its wall whatever of the chyle is necessary for its own nutrition. The remainder is conveyed by veins to the liver, there to be further refined and converted into blood for the nourishment of the rest of the body. To Galen, it would seem, this meant that all digestion occurs in the stomach and liver, with the remainder of the intestinal tract functioning essentially as a conduit for eliminating wastes. But like most other scripture, Galen's writings contain contradictions. He goes on to say that some of the coction continues in the intestine, with the chyle resulting from this later phase being carried to the liver by the veins lying along the intestine's many feet of length. Like Galen's teachings in anatomy, his formulation of digestion remained, in its complete or a modified form, a dominating force in the minds of physicians until the late Renaissance. Some of his other doctrines persisted for centuries beyond even that time.

It would be impossible to overestimate Galen's monarchical dominance over medical thought, for well more than a millennium and a half after his death in 201 C.E. He was the authority to whom all physicians turned; he was the idol who would have to be shattered before scientific medicine could begin its long journey toward today. Although his formulations would be modified over the centuries, few physicians dared question their all-encompassing theoretical basis. His heritage was a huge oeuvre and an equally huge reputation for infallibility. The great men of medieval and early Renaissance medicine were no more than redactors and commentators on Galen.

How did one man become such an icon of healing that his every word reverberated down the centuries? Galen, a Greek born in

Pergamon, Asia Minor, in 131 C.E., was the most skilled physician of his time and a voluminous writer. If published in a modern edition, his extant works would occupy more than 20 thick octavo volumes of closely printed material. Though a uniquely accomplished experimenter, he was nevertheless a typical Greek thinker to whom philosophical speculations and the employment of logic were just as valid—if not more so—as unbiased observation. His teachings are characterized by an unfailing disposition to fill in the gaps between things which were known with things which were not. Galen's speculations arose from a convinced application of the theory of humors and the equally convinced thesis that an omniscient supreme intellect had not only created a grand design of nature in which every structure displayed a perfection of function and purpose but had also superintended every detail of its construction.

Galen's writings are filled with declarations of his superiority over all rivals and disdain for those without his self-proclaimed medical certainty. He rose to great heights of fame in Rome, eventually becoming personal physician to the emperor, Marcus Aurelius. Most of his authority derived from his indubitable contributions as an experimenter on animals as well as his writings and extensive lecturing. His air of infallibility and an unquestioning acceptance by his contemporaries were such that his theories became the basis of medical dogma, and remained so for dozens of generations.

Though hypothetical, Galen's was the earliest systematic explanation for the stomach's role in the maintenance of life. While steadfastly denying any possibility of moment-to-moment supernatural intervention, he was nevertheless convinced that human anatomy and function were created by a process of divine architecture and a specific plan mediated through the power he called Nature. In that plan, he saw only perfection. To him, everything was ideally made and supremely suited for the role assigned to it. He seems also to have believed in a single god, whom he saw as the artisan responsible for having made all living things from materials in existence before the creation of the world: "You should see that every part performs its different, well-tempered action by the aid of a suitable construction; that the Creator has bestowed upon each one certain godlike faculties."

In the Galenic scheme, there appears to have been no chemical component to the process of coction. Like his followers for many centuries after him, Galen believed that the stomach does its work by the compressive action of the powerful sheets of muscle fibers he saw in its wall. He likened the process to the pressing of wine from grapes, and believed it to be modified by an innate heat which he thought to be a property of the stomach. In keeping with humoral theory, the source of the innate heat was the heart. The dregs resulting from coction, he taught, sink to the bottom of the stomach and toward the bowel, while the chyle rises, "bubbling and fermenting like new wine from the heart of the viscus."

Long before Galen and long after him, it was believed that there was some intrinsic power within the stomach that accounts for its ability to digest food. So vaguely defined was this power that it was not susceptible to any kind of analysis of its quantity or nature. Neither fluid nor solid, it was rather an ability consistent with the general thesis that would in later centuries become known as vitalism—the notion that some unknowable vital force or energy exists within living things that pervades all parts of an organism, gives it life, and permits it to function. Vitalism ran like a consistent thread through the patterns of medical thought until late in the nineteenth century, and even now appears in various forms as part of certain alternative and traditional healing methods. This mysterious force was thought to manifest itself in a variety of ways. Some theoreticians were convinced that it imparts to each organ its own distinctive potency in the life of the total creature.

In noting the centrality and even authority of the stomach, Galen was continuing in a venerable tradition. So old is that tradition that a genre of fable exists concerning the stomach, fragments of which have been found dating as far back as 1100 B.C.E. In a typical example, one or all of the other organs rise up against the stomach's authority, as citizens might attempt to cast off the yoke of the head of state. It is specifically this story that is told as a cautionary tale by the patrician Menenius Agrippa in the opening scene of Shakespeare's *Coriolanus,* as he tries to dissuade a group of armed and mutinous plebeians determined to revolt against the overweening power of the Roman nobility. In an analogy with the dominance of the state, Menenius quotes the stomach describing the other organs' dependency on it:

> The strongest nerves and small inferior veins
> From me receive that natural competency
> Whereby they live:

and compares the stomach to:

> The helms o' the state, who care for you like fathers,
> When you curse them as enemies.

Menenius warns the plebeians of the futility of rebellion against such authority, whether it be governmental or gastric:

> [Y]ou may as well
> Strike at the heaven with your staves as lift them
> Against the Roman state;

Like other of Shakespeare's plot devices, this one is based on fact. According to Roman historians, a patrician named Menenius Agrippa did indeed prevent a rebellion of plebeian secessionists in 494 B.C.E. by telling them this fable. Having done so, he proceeded to the moral, epitomized in what are said to have been his closing words: "You see, then, that the senate in the State is what the stomach is in the body . . . In the same way, the senate rules the common weal and provides what appertains to each part whereby it saves them all from destruction."

The German historian Walter Pagel, who calls such tales *stomachus in fabula,* notes how common they were, and that they are "a variation on a perennial theme that has attracted fabulists from ancient Egyptian times to the nineteenth century. Their basic story belongs to the stock-in-trade of the ancient, medieval and modern fable-literature which extended from India to the Middle East and Western Europe." Everywhere, it seems, the stomach has been recognized for its lordly character.

As Galen himself pointed out, the upper portion of the stomach had long before his time been called the cardia, because it is near the heart and is therefore its close companion and the source for some of its qualities. The ancient Egyptian word for stomach, in fact, means "mouth of the heart."

By Galen's time, a notion known as sympathy had been in existence for centuries: Changes in certain organs affect the behavior of one or more of their fellows, as though there were some form of communion between them, due either to proximity or the mediation by special vessels of otherwise undefined nature, connecting one to the other. In Roman times, some of the emotions, especially those of the sensitive sort that can cause moodiness, gloom, or wrath, were thought to originate in the stomach and only secondarily to manifest themselves in the heart. Effects now known to be due to nerve impulses and blood-borne chemical messengers were until the fairly recent past thought to be the result of such "sympathy," the word John Abernethy used in the early nineteenth century to describe the relationship between digestion and the nervous system.

The sympathy thought to exist between cardia and cardiac—the upper stomach and the heart—is the reason that symptoms originating in one were often attributed to the other. To this day, we speak of "heartburn" when what is really meant is the discomfort caused by acid stomach contents regurgitating up into the lowest part of the esophagus, or food-pipe. There is thus an intermingling of terms and characteristics of the two organs. Moreover, the esophagus and the heart being anatomically so close, the need to differentiate between the two as the site of discomfort was thought to be of little consequence.

There is thus an intermingling not only in terminology and putative characteristics but even of the locations of the two organs. Especially did the emotional or personality factors attributed primarily to one become associated with the other. For those who believed, as did Aristotle, that the heart is the seat of the mind, it was hardly a leap to conclude that the stomach as well played a major role in the passions and in thought. "Not having the heart for it" is very close (although nowadays sometimes used just a bit differently) to "not having the stomach for it." As recently as the mid-nineteenth century, the anatomical term *precordium* was defined in two distinct ways by medical dictionaries—as the area of the chest in front of the heart, and separately as the uppermost portion of the central abdomen, lying a bit lower than the breastbone. Today, the word refers only to the former.

The characteristics thought to reside in the diaphragm display a similar pattern. That broad sheet of muscle, lying as it does between stomach and heart and in direct contact with both, was caught up in the same mythology of emotions and thought as its two neighbors and was long believed to have absorbed their characteristics. The synonym used by anatomists and physicians for diaphragmatic (from the Greek *diaphragma*, meaning "a partition") has always been *phrenic*, derived from the Greek plural *phrenes*, meaning "the muscular diaphragm." The singular, *phren*, means "the mind," or "the seat of the emotions." Because of its continuity with both the heart and the cardia of the stomach, the diaphragm, or *phrenes*, had from pre-Homeric times half a millennium before Hippocrates been regarded by the Greeks as the seat of reason. From these connotations are derived such words as *frenetic* and *schizophrenic*. Phrenology, the discredited pseudoscience that analyzes a person's character by studying the bumps on his head, derives from the same source.

There is a vagueness and overlapping in all of this, reflecting the ancient uncertainty and disagreement about just which of the two, heart or stomach, is predominant in its control over the rest of the body and of so much of the processes of emotion and thought. The stomach's ascendancy in the hierarchy faded rapidly during the Middle Ages, so that by the Renaissance its previous lordliness had long been forgotten, replaced, not surprisingly, by those of the heart and the brain. Nevertheless, isolated examples are to be found right up through that period, of physicians who continued to exalt it. In his monumental 1314 text, *Chirurgie*, the French surgeon Henri de Mondeville called the stomach "the most principal and the most noble membre in the body." The fifteenth-century Italian anatomist Alessandro Benedetti thought of it as "the father of the family," believing that it controlled the integrity of the entire living creature. But such statements are rare after the early medieval period. Most authors saw the stomach as an organ the importance of whose function meant that its neighbors must take care of it.

The predominant Renaissance view of the stomach seems to have derived from a combination of its location and its supposed sympathetic response to the structures near it. From each of them, it took on characteristics that determine its temperament. The stomach's great importance to digestion was said to assure that all of the organ's neighbors recognized that its centrality of position reflected the centrality of its needs, which they were obliged to fulfill. This viewpoint is epitomized in the following passage from a 1577 treatise written by the anatomist Thomas Vicary, the first Master of the United Company of Barbers and Surgeons of England:

> It hath the lyver on the right side, chafing & heating him with his lobes or figures: & the Splen on the left syde, with his fatnes, and veynes sending to him melancholie, to exercise his appetites: and above him is the Harte, quickening him with his Arteries: Also the Brayne, send to him a braunch of Nerves to geve him feeling.

Finally, as though to prove the point that intellectual *tabulae rasae* and new paradigms of conjecture are the exception—and the rare exception at that—rather than the rule in human thought, supremacy was returned to the stomach in the early seventeenth century writings of a remarkably productive if somewhat mercurial Belgian physician, Jean Baptiste van Helmont, who insisted that he was presenting an original thesis.

Van Helmont was a perennially troubled and confused man, who, while a Capuchin monk in Louvain, had experienced apocalyptic visions involving his guardian angel, St. Raphael, that turned him to the intensive study of the writings of Hippocrates, Galen, and a first-century C.E. medical botanist named Dioscorides. One can only speculate about why a man of the cloth should choose to bury himself in the works of ancient physicians, but it is worth noting a fact probably known to him: *Raphael* is Hebrew for "healer of God."

Although he became a physician as a result of his obsessional immersion in the ancient works, van Helmont seems never to have made up his mind whether an understanding of human physiology is better discovered in experimental studies or in mystical thinking. His formulations, and in fact his life, are somewhat like a pendulum of uncertainty, swinging back and forth between science and mysticism. But unlike the predictably harmonic motion of pendulums, he seems in the main to have swung his arc in fits and starts, and often to have lingered too long in the middle. In this, he may be seen as a man characteristic of his age, in which deduction from synthesized all-explanatory theories and the recently introduced principles of inductive reasoning lived side by side with the old patterns of superstition and religious belief. But the oscillations of his mind were so feverish and his thinking so imbued with pure make-believe that he exemplified his age writ large, with its worst inconsistencies in bold relief. Not content to believe only what he could prove, he insisted, like the Greeks and every other school of thought before him, on introducing nonmaterial factors into his speculative explanations. Specifically, he believed that experimental demonstrations and logic were limited in their ability to reveal truth. "Real knowledge," he wrote, "must by its very nature involve intuition." To van Helmont, intuition meant inspiration by spiritually based imaginings. From this conviction arose his stomach-centered theory of human biology, compounded of science, orthodox religious principles, and magic. That the three make strange bedfellows is illustrated in the next chapter, by the story of his misguided search for truth.

CHAPTER THREE

THE STOMACH:

GHOSTLY GASES,

MYSTICAL ACIDS

T HE irony of Jean Baptiste van Helmont's erroneous claim to priority with regard to the stomach's centrality is that his formulations did indeed arise out of an entirely new theme, which he introduced into serious medical thought—a concept that became known as iatrochemistry (*iatros,* the Greek word for "healer" or "physician"). The underlying precepts of iatrochemistry had recently been formulated by an innovative Swiss thinker named Paracelsus, who lived in the early decades of the sixteenth century. But Paracelsus was a personality even more erratic than van Helmont, and his controversial reputation inhibited easy adoption of his ideas. It was the research and theorizing of van Helmont that secured the position in medical theory of this startling new thesis: All life is the result of chemical processes.

But for van Helmont, it was not enough to do the experiments and demonstrate the evidence upon which such a revolutionary idea achieved acceptance. He had to go further. Like the Greeks and virtually all other theoreticians who preceded him, van Helmont felt called upon to present a theory that would explain the functioning of all living things, and indeed of the universe. Nothing would do but that he should provide a total explanation of the biological events he studied, and divine factors had to be at its core.

It was van Helmont's contention that each of the body's chemical processes is controlled by a specific guiding agent. Requiring a term for these agents, he invented the word *gas,* which he derived from *chaos,* the ancient Greek term for the nebulous space in which was contained the unformed mass of basic substances in existence before the creation of the universe. As he saw it, each object or type of matter has its own gas, and it is this gas which gives it specificity. The blood, for example, lives because of its specific and unique gas, which bears the determinants of its formation and function.

Not yet content with the degree to which he was testing credulity, van Helmont tortured the concept into its next stage, stating that the gas is not contained *in* the object but actually *is* the object without its original shape or form. This can be proven, he claimed, by distilling or heating the structure or fluid, whereupon it is converted into a vapor, which is its pure essence and its gas—absent the material's outward shape. It is still matter, but it is not *really* matter, for the gas is a spiritual thing. The implication of this is that the behavior of every substance in nature is unique unto itself and determined by its own distinctive organization, of which its gas is the basis. Each gas is supervised by a special spirit, or *archeus,* a word derived from the Greek *arche,* referring to a first principle. Thus, although van Helmont is correctly credited as the discoverer of "gas," he used the word with implications far beyond its present meaning.

The notion of archeus had been introduced into medicine by Paracelsus, who believed that each of the four elements of Empedocles—earth, air, fire, and water—contains an active principle that gives life to dead matter. He called this principle the archeus. Long before Paracelsus, this concept of an inscrutable and quite hypothetical vital force—vitalism—had pervaded the thinking of many of the researchers and philosophers who tried to explain the nature of living things. Oswald Croll, one of Paracelsus's leading disciples, gave about as clear a description of his teacher's ideas on such matters as can be found, when he wrote in 1609 of "the archeus of man, or internal chemist, born within and implanted by God." Though later vitalists did not necessarily invoke God, they believed nevertheless in a force beyond the ability of physics and chemistry to explain.

In hypothesizing an immaterial spirit guiding in some way a factor real or at least thought to be real, van Helmont was following another old tradition, whose origins go as far back as the fifth or sixth Egyptian dynasties and are traceable until the thirtieth, and then forward into Europe to the Middle Ages. The Egyptians believed that every organ of the body was watched over by its own god or goddess. A number of papyri exist from various periods in which each organ is listed. Most of the lists end with the phrase "There is no part of the body without its god." In similar fashion, during the Middle Ages the individual parts of the body were said to be protected by the individual signs of the zodiac. In such ways, the microcosm and the macrocosm are united.

But van Helmont, as the product of sixteen centuries of Christianity's unquestioning belief in the primacy of the soul over all else in a person, felt justified in going even further. The various archei, he claimed, function under the general control of something that is indeed a soul. According to him, the soul is a motivating spiritual quality located in the cardia of the stomach, from which its influence diffuses throughout the body. In this way, the spiritual principle that is the archeus can act autonomously at the same time that it is integrated harmoniously into the life-giving principle of the entire person. Disease is an alteration of this supreme archeus, and death is its loss. In all of his formulations, van Helmont claimed to be inspired by God, the source of the quality he called intuition. If so, God's inspired message about the location of the soul must have been garbled in transmission, because van Helmont's explanation for it was more than a little peculiar: His thesis was based on the observation that a hard blow in the "pit of the stomach" eliminates consciousness.

Modern historians search the writings of colleagues and those from other disciplines for the cardinal sin of what they call presentism—judging events or people of the past by the standards or knowledge of today. But even the most self-righteous of such critics would be hard put to accuse a skeptic of miscreance when he points out the obvious ludicrousness of van Helmont's anatomic justification. Consciousness is much more effectively destroyed by hitting a man over the head than by aiming for his belly. Why then did he not locate the soul within the skull? Was it because others, whom van Helmont considered on a lower intellectual level than himself, had been doing so for centuries? Had he been more pugilistically oriented, would he have placed it in the jaw?

By the period during which van Helmont lived, it had long been recognized as undeniable that the brain is involved in thought processes. To deal with that bothersome reality, he replied that the brain, though important, is secondary to the stomach. His God-inspired logic made the brain an intermediary between the stomach and the rest of the body, because it is connected to both by nerves. He assigned to the brain the faculties of memory and imagination (to the heart was given free will), but the quality of understanding—considered by him to be the essence of the mind—could come only from the stomach, since he would brook no disagreement with his assertion that it was indisputably the mind's seat.

The fact is that van Helmont's contention that the soul and mind are located in the stomach was the result of an insight gained while he was under the influence of a poison called wolfsbane, the active ingredient of which has since been determined to be the drug aconitine, one of whose most prominent actions is to cause mental confusion. Tingling, warmth, and convulsions are also common, all effects that divinely inspired seers have at times experienced since men began keeping records of such things. Van Helmont had ingested the wolfsbane as part of an experiment he was conducting at the time, based on his conviction that poisons contain what he called virgin powers. Shortly after taking it, he sensed that something in his upper abdomen was controlling his perception and understanding of things around him. This realization came to him in a form he later described as being remarkably pleasant and lucid. His description brings to mind the many tales of hallucinogen-induced wisdom that have been current in our own era (perhaps *especially* in our own era) and fits remarkably closely with the state of mind reported by those who have returned from what are called near-death experiences.

Despite its supernal entanglements, van Helmont's emphasis on the primacy of chemical events in biological processes paved the way for other, more objective, researchers to build on his teachings. Whatever its misdirection, his contribution that gases are entities distinct from air ("Gas is a far more subtle or fine thing than a vapour, mist or distilled oylinesses, although as yet it be many times thicker than air") was absolutely seminal in later work, for which he himself laid the groundwork by discovering carbon dioxide. Still, so enmeshed in mystical meanings were his writings about this gas (which he derived by allowing acetic acid to act on calcium carbonate—vinegar on chalk), that it had to be rediscovered in 1757 by an English chemist, Joseph Black.

Van Helmont's resort to the hypothetical archeus and the equally hypothetical qualities he attributed to gases is exemplary of that perennial human trait of inventing what cannot be observed—a mixture of the supernatural and the imaginary—to fill in the gaps and voids between what is verifiable and what is needed to complete the substantiation of a worldview. We seek out what is missing, and make it up when it cannot be found. The hallmark of these patterns is the manufacture of vaguely expressed and even more vaguely understood "facts" to justify a preconceived all-explanatory theory or philosophy. The facts not being facts, they are sometimes inconsistent with one another or open to fuzzy interpretations. The entire edifice is thus supported on a vague and often internally contradictory framework that in time may develop a flexible and polymorphic logic of its own, accepted by similarly predisposed adherents whose standards for accepting "evidence" is lax. Millennia ago, men created elves and goblins; more recently, they have been visited by angels or cure disease by influencing the flow of vital energies. As so trenchantly said of van Helmont himself by the historian Arturo Castiglioni, "His explanations of different archaei . . . not only explained nothing, but did not even seem clear in the mind of their author."

Sometimes such mystical schemata become the accepted wisdom of a movement or even a large segment of the population. Living on for generation after generation, they may eventually enter the unchallenged tradition of an entire people—becoming a part of their identity—who never subject them to the trial of experiment or logical reasoning. Even when science has provided chemical and physical explanations, these may be unknown or ignored by adherents of the old concepts. In more recent times, such scientific explanations have sometimes even been rejected as representing the constricting views of an oppressive elite. In the minds of the supporters of received beliefs—such as the theories of healing called "traditional medicine"—to question them is to question the values of a society or of a group of committed believers. Worse yet, the scrutiny of scientific skepticism, when it is applied to such systems, is perceived as an expression of the cultural or intellectual arrogance of outsiders who seek to impose their own values or approach to knowledge. These responses tie the hands of those who would simply seek truth. The resistance makes it impossible to extract any nuggets of demonstrable worth from systems whose generalized philosophies may in other ways be flawed. Were it otherwise, alternative healing practices would be studied by scientists much more thoroughly than they are.

In his own time there were far fewer thinkers equipped to challenge van Helmont than would exist only a century later. In fact, there were probably none. In his formulations, the stomach became not only supreme once again but, as might be expected of the seat of the soul, it took its place as the source of an entire range of thoughts and emotions. Van Helmont arrived at these notions by "intuition," a process of whose validity he was convinced. His "intuition," for example informed him that the stomach's outlet, the pylorus, is subject to the same emotions as any living animal. It has knowledge, he claimed, of what is in the interests of the body, and acts accordingly. When bad food reaches it, the pylorus "judges" (*censet,* in his Latin) that the body would be harmed by it. To prevent this, it shuts down tightly and sends a wave of motion backward in the stomach toward the esophagus, resulting in vomiting. It does this because it "knows" what is right. In addition, the pylorus feels "indignation" when it senses poison in the stomach and sets off responses that induce a paralysis of the body. Or it may be "furious" when some remote structure, such as an arm, is injured. In its state of fury, it will induce vomiting, which will not cease until the limb is treated. This occurs because an organ's archeus has psychic powers. It can act on other structures of the body—it becomes the agent of "sympathy."

Van Helmont's conviction of the validity of intuition is in itself instructive. Proponents of mistaken systems then and now have only in rare cases been fraudulent. Their errors have in the main been made by underestimating the standards upon which real evidence must be based. Often, the drawing of false conclusions is simply a matter of the human propensity to resort to a confidence in *post hoc* reasoning: *post hoc, ergo propter hoc* ("after this, therefore because of this"). Another common fallacy is insufficient differentiation between subjective and objective. Related to and frequently following from this kind of fuzziness is the failure to appreciate that mere impressions (or sometimes wishful thinking) do not have the same validity as those observations that can be tested repeatedly with one's five senses and reproduced in the detached experience of others. To theorists who speculate in these questionable ways, in fact, the sixth sense carries more weight than the other five combined.

Such errors in logic are obvious to us today, but they were hardly so in van Helmont's time. It was only with the major advances in science and experimental research which became plentiful long after his death that the rules of evidence and the necessity for detached observations free of preconception became apparent. Contemporary thought permitted speculations of the sort proposed by van Helmont, especially when they could be justified as consistent with the religious belief that was universal throughout Europe and unquestioned as the source of all being. It is difficult, perhaps, for the modern mind to conceive of a science in thrall to theological dogma, but everything we know of the study of nature until at least the eighteenth century must be interpreted in the light of that indisputable state of subservience. As so aptly put in 1930 by the historian of embryology F. J. Cole, "To science was allotted the subordinate role of providing the material demonstration of the Divine Plan." When van Helmont wrote of archei, intuition, and soul, he was doing just that. Though we may be tempted to criticize his formulations for going beyond what was considered necessary for his church-dominated time, he was convinced that even the most far-fetched of his theories were divinely inspired. He lived when he lived, and not today. It is when mystical explanations and unverifiable observations are used as evidence in our own time— when we know better—that the protests of reasonable people are not only justified but required.

Its questionable mix notwithstanding, van Helmont's philosophy bore within itself the seeds of its own destruction. By introducing chemical principles into the study of physiology, van Helmont did help to bring about a more science-based understanding of how our bodies work—one that would in time overthrow his own "intuitive" model.

Van Helmont's melange of scientific and nonscientific principles is exemplified by his views on digestion. In his day, the accepted understanding of digestion was still one or another variation on the principle of coction, the formulation received from Galen, in which the ingested food was ground up by the stomach and cooked by that organ's innate heat, much as one would prepare soup or stew from meat, vegetables, and water. Although several different theories existed, each emphasizing its own aspect of the process, all took the essential characteristics of coction to be accurate. Having conducted experiments in which he identified the presence of acid in the stomach of pigeons, van Helmont did not hesitate to state that acid is the major factor in the digestive processes of all animals. For this remarkable insight, he deserves to be recognized as the discoverer of the principle of acid gastric digestion. But he was not satisfied to limit his theorizing to the kind of speculation that is justifiable on the basis of a real set of reproducible observations. Here, too, he added some vitalism—just enough to inhibit further attempts at investigating the ways in which the acid actually acts on food. With no experimental observations to support him, he declared that the acid does not do the digesting itself but acts on an invisible quality or spirit called a ferment, which in some undefined way does the job. In other words, the acid was more than just an acid—it had an archeuslike ferment that caused the process to take place. In this, van Helmont was borrowing from the alchemists, to whom a ferment was a nonmaterial spiritual agent that had the power to convert one substance into another.

Although his views on some matters were derived from such a conjunction of science and mysticism, other ideas came even more directly from van Helmont's devout religious convictions. He convinced himself, for example, that all physical bodies are ultimately reducible to water, which he considered the only pure form of matter. The hypothesis that everything physical consists in the last resort of water was the result of his unquestioning acceptance of an interpretation of Genesis 1:2, agreed upon by many theologians of the time: "And the spirit of God moved upon the face of the waters." The faithful took this to mean that water is older and therefore more fundamental than earth.

Even here van Helmont mixed the spiritual and what might be called the scientific, or at least a theory that has some basis in observation. According to Aristotle, the notion that water is the substance from which all other matter is made originated with the sixth-century B.C.E. Greek philosopher Thales. Apparently, Thales's observation that water not only moves but can change itself into vapor convinced him that it was the closest of all substances to life itself. In fact, life cannot exist without it. To Thales, this meant not only that water is the ulti-· mate substance, but that the living organism which is the entire universe is sustained by it. Like living things, water, he believed, possesses psyche, the animating principle.

But here again, van Helmont insisted on going further, finally taking the hypothesis well beyond the point where the theologians had been content to leave it. Determined to provide an experimental proof to bolster his belief system, he planted a willow tree of known weight and nourished it with nothing but water for five years. At the end of that time, it had grown considerably, gaining a total of 164 pounds. To van Helmont, the evidence was indisputable that all the tree's new substance was made of water: "164 pounds of Wood, Barks and Roots arose out of water onely." What is even more remarkable than his specious reasoning is that many of the leading thinkers of the time accepted his statement, based as it was on "experimental evidence." The fact that the "evidence" was misinterpreted seems not to have been appreciated, and this too is a lesson for our time. The loud, clear voice with which authority so often proclaims itself has ever been a danger to the pursuit of truth. The fact that we know better today has not yet freed us from the dictates of authority.

With the increasing emphasis on chemical researches that occurred later in the seventeenth century, a more balanced viewpoint about how the various organs contribute to the economy of the entire body began after a time to come into focus. The notion of organs as individual personalities or autonomous city-states within the national structure; the distinctive lordliness or subordinate position of one or another body part; the search for sources of the soul or the animating spirit—all of these would gradually give way during the following era, in the face of a determined effort by a relatively few investigators to reduce all natural factors to the fundamental principles of chemistry and physics.

But before it was understood that the answers must be sought in chemistry *and* physics, a great deal of activity was expended by researchers determined to prove that the proper direction was one or the other, but not both. During van Helmont's time and later, the metaphor of the body as teeming laboratory of chemical interactions was defended with a vigor bordering on fanaticism against the metaphor of the body as structural machine. Truth be told, these were, in fact, hardly metaphors. They were taken quite literally by their respective exponents. Two competing schools of thought grew up around these disagreements, becoming known as the iatrophysicists (some of them might better be called iatromathematicians) and the iatrochemists, the founding father of whom was van Helmont himself. So determined was each group to achieve ascendancy that neither of them hesitated to invent complicated and abstruse systems relying on mechanics and mathematics on the one hand and the emerging findings of chemistry mixed with a modified form of alchemy on the other in order to advance their respective causes.

Even the most prominent philosopher of the age joined in the fray. René Descartes expounded his views on natural law by insisting that the body is a machine that operates under the guidance of a rational soul, which he located in the pineal gland, at the base of the brain. Since the soul is single and distinctive, he reasoned, it must make its home in the one structure of the body he believed to fulfill the same criteria while also being anatomically close to the brain. (He seems not to have taken into account the pituitary gland, described by Galen.) Enough of Galen remained in Descartes's thinking that he ascribed the movements of the heart to its innate heat, as though it were some source of internal fire providing energy for the workings of the machinery.

If van Helmont represents the ultimate in iatrochemistry, then surely the mechanical view was epitomized in the writings of one Giorgio Baglivi of Rome, who went so far as to divide the human machine into innumerable smaller machines. In his magnum opus of 1704, *Opera omnia medico-practica et anatomica,* Baglivi described the fundamentals of his thesis, while figuratively in the same breath decrying the arguments of his opponents: "Whoever examines the bodily organism with attention will certainly not fail to discern pincers in the jaws and teeth; a container in the stomach; water-mains in the veins, the arteries and the other ducts; a piston in the heart; sieves or filters in the bowels; in the lungs, bellows; in the muscles, the force of the lever; in the corner of the eye, a pulley, and so on. So let the chemists continue to explain natural phenomena in complex terms such as fusion, sublimation, precipitation, etc., thus founding a separate philosophy. It remains unquestionable that all these phenomena must be seen in the forces of the wedge, of equilibrium, of the lever, of the spring, and of all the other principles of mechanics. In short, the natural functions of the living body can be explained in no other way so clearly and easily as by means of the experimental and mathematical principles with which nature herself speaks."

Some of Baglivi's fellow mechanists went beyond even such categorizations. The Neapolitan mathematician Giovanni Borelli somehow calculated that one of the muscles flexing the thumb, the flexor pollicis longus, was capable of producing a pulling force of 3,720 pounds. Since the flexor weighs two ounces, it was reasoned that each ounce of any muscle or muscular organ is able to exert a force of about 1,800 pounds. Other like-minded iatrophysicists, on finding the stomach to weigh some eight ounces, pronounced its compressive force to be truly enormous (an Englishman named Pitcairn estimated it to be 12,951 pounds!). This calculation supported Borelli's thesis that the organ does its job by pulverizing ingested food, which can then be acted upon by a corrosive juice like that which he had found in the stomach of dolphins. The iatrophysicists were chagrined when later researchers, doing direct experiments, discovered that the stomach would burst at relatively low pressures. Van Helmont had gone off in the other direction, inventing (and "inventing" is the only word for it) six different ferments to account for his unsubstantiated theory that there are six sequential stages of digestion.

In the next century, the virulent disagreements between the iatrophysicists and iatrochemists would be held up to scorn. John Hunter, the outspoken Scottish researcher who is single-handedly responsible for introducing the experimental approach into surgery, had his own words of ridicule for the many analogies of which each camp was so fond: In 1784, he told an audience of physicians in London, "Some physiologists will have it, that the stomach is a mill, others, that it is a fermenting vat, others again, that it is a stew-pan; but, in my view of the matter, it is neither a mill, a fermenting vat nor a stew-pan; but a stomach, gentlemen, a stomach."

Even in the face of his erroneous conceptions, Baglivi, like van Helmont, pursued laboratory studies that had important consequences for future researchers to build upon. In 1700, he was the first to distinguish between voluntary (or striped) and involuntary (or smooth) muscle fibers. The one factor uniting iatrochemists and iatrophysicists was their mutual inability to explain observed phenomena without resorting to the invocation of forces and energies whose existence was purely speculative, which is a charitable way to say imaginary. Though clothed in the language of mechanics and chemistry—bellows, waterworks, heat, ferments, gas—both sides ultimately attributed primary power to unknowable vitalistic qualities, such as an archeus. To some, like van Helmont, these qualities were God-given; to a gradually increasing number of others, they were a property of nature, which further studies might one day elucidate.

Not having rid themselves of the ages-old certainty that inscrutable powers are everywhere—formerly sprites, elves, and gods; now an archeus, ferments, gases, and "life forces"—many medical theorists up through the late nineteenth century injected, far more than some of them realized, vitalist and spiritual beliefs into their chemical or physical speculations. Even the renowned Sir Francis Bacon, who wrote so convincingly of the value of inductive reasoning that he is commonly regarded as having introduced the patterns of modern experimental science, was not innocent of invoking "spirits" to explain phenomena for which he could not otherwise account. His writings are filled with examples of this, from spirits in the brain and muscles that move the body to those that facilitate vision. John Hunter, too, that greatest of all eighteenth-century surgeons (and a master of detached observation), spoke of an innate property he called the living principle, a vitalistic force animating all creatures and giving them life. To the agnostic Hunter, this was an as yet unknown, nature-derived factor.

The iatrochemists believed *they* had freed themselves of supernaturalism because they studied the actions of real materials, such as acids, digestive juices, and those gases that could be produced in the laboratory; the iatrophysicists believed *they* had rid themselves of supernaturalism because they utilized mathematical and physical principles similar to those employed by such eminent scientists as Galileo, Newton, Pascal, and Leibniz. Out of this inchoate agglomeration of fact and fancy would come the medical science of the next era.

By the final third of the eighteenth century, the most productive of the medical theorists were beginning to realize that their aims must be more limited. They had come to accept that it was not necessary to provide all-inclusive explanations for the vast array of the phenomena of life. It was becoming clear, in fact, that the most direct path toward comprehensive understanding was the straightforward one of making repeated observations of relatively localized phenomena without attempting to put them together into a hypothesis until some reasonable pattern became evident. Gradually discarded was the old approach of introducing a grand theory to elucidate the totality of all biology and then invoking imaginary factors to fill in the empty spaces. As John Hunter would say of medicine, it is "from the depths, not from the heights, that medicine is fed; from the springs, not from the sky." No longer would it be considered within the province of science to seek for primary instigators. If there was a single element that contributed most to the rise of scientific medicine, it was this: Researchers no longer expected that they should understand nature through some universally explanatory scheme.

The paradox of the situation is remarkable: so long as hardly *anything* was known about the basis of human biology, theorists tried to explain *everything*. Once real knowledge began to increase by the progressive discovery of facts verifiable by instruments or in the laboratory, objectives became more realistically modest. The impulse to reach far into imagination for nonmaterial answers to elucidate the mysteries of biology and the cosmos lessened concomitantly with the advent of reproducible experimental studies directed toward specific and quite limited problems. Ironically, now at the turn of the twenty-first century, one result of working "from the springs, not the sky" has been that science once again finds itself concerned with what is being called a theory of everything—the so-called great universal theory—and the fulfillment of that ancient quest may in fact be visible on the horizon. But more about that later.

The new "from the depths" thinking had far-reaching effects on research aimed at explaining the functions of the stomach, as exemplified in a series of experiments carried out by René Réaumur, a French naturalist so independently wealthy that he devoted much of his life to studying various problems that chanced to excite his curiosity. Apparently fed up (pun intended) with the fanciful characteristics his contemporaries were attributing to the acid that was being identified in the stomachs of various animals, and unconvinced that the exponents of pulverization were providing more than a small part of the explanation for digestion, he designed a study to determine once and for all whether the significant factor was or was not chemical.

Réaumur had a pet kite, a bird of the hawk family. Such an animal regurgitates from its stomach all material that is indigestible, which in 1752 gave its inventive owner the idea of feeding the creature by putting food into small metallic tubes whose ends were covered by wire gratings, so that any surrounding liquid might easily find its way inside. When the kite predictably puked up the tubes, much of the food was found to be digested, even though there was no possibility that any compressive action of the gastric wall could have affected it through the rigid metal casing. Convinced that the bitter fluid he found within the tubes was acid, he repeated the experiments, but this time he replaced the food with sponges to suck up the liquid substance. After the kite regurgitated the indigestible meal, he squeezed the sponges out and found that the retrieved fluid turned blue litmus paper pink, and thereby convinced himself that the active factor in gastric digestion is indeed acid. The evidence was clear and seemed to obviate the need to dream up hypothetical spirits or anima. Réaumur went so far as to incubate the acid with bits of meat, noting that at room temperature the digestion was incomplete. As would the American physician William Beaumont seventy years later, he interpreted this to mean that the completion of the process required a temperature approximating that of the body. It was just at this point that Réaumur's kite had the bad grace to die. When continuing his studies using dogs and sheep proved unsatisfactory, the intellectually restless amateur naturalist drifted toward other matters. He finally abandoned his studies, never to take them up again.

It might be thought that Réaumur's carefully designed experiments would make some lasting impression on the vitalists and seekers after ineffable spiritual forces. It was not to be. Close though it may have been, the time had not yet arrived for observations to be taken at face value without the necessity by certain resistant men to look for something deeper, or rather something more lofty. The makers of speculative systems simply pointed out that the kite was a living thing and therefore carried in its gastric juices the vitalizing and quite unknowable forces by which all organic activities are explainable. These were, after all, men of a mind with those who were convinced that wine ferments because it carries the inscrutable force that gave life to the grape from which it was pressed.

But the time was nearing when primary instigators would less often be sought in the realm of supernature and more often in the direct effects of chemistry and physics. The transition would be gradual, and to this day it remains incomplete. In the minds of much of mankind, everyday events still seem easier to understand if they are seen as part of a sometimes predetermined and sometimes capricious pattern, in the hands of nonmaterial powers. But progress toward real understanding has never been made by believing in such supernal modes. It was only with this new thinking that the magnificent accomplishments of twentieth-century science were possible.

Just as the story of the stomach provides an epitome of the old ways and their reliance on forces beyond human ken, it elucidates also the progressive turning to modern scientific precepts. The new thinking affected mankind's understanding of the stomach in ways impossible to have imagined before it supplanted the old. It would at first clarify the essentially chemical nature of gastric digestion and put its mechanical aspects into perspective; it would then permit productive study of diseases of the stomach like ulcer and cancer; it would in time find treatments for those diseases, incorporating medical means and surgery; it would go on to investigate the effects of hormones, other signaling molecules, and neurological factors on the stomach; it would develop ways to study the inside of the digestive tract using lighted, camera-bearing flexible tubes as well as imaging techniques like X ray; it would, in our time, utilize the new findings in molecular biology to elucidate the nature of the active transport of acid into the gastric cavity, by pumping, through the cells lining the stomach's inner wall.

As in any journey, there were periods of fascinating outbursts of progress, periods of slow, hard slogging, and periods even of misdirected efforts. A profusion of names, experimental studies, and theories were to appear. Several of the most prominent deserve attention, because each of them was a first in a series of discoveries that have transformed our image—literally and figuratively—not only of the stomach's physiological functions but also of its interactions with the man or woman in whom it dwells and even with their thoughts and the events of their lives.

Scarcely more than a year after Wilhelm Conrad Röntgen of the University of Würzburg discovered X rays on a fateful Friday evening in November 1895, two Harvard medical students began experimenting with the new technology to study the swallowing mechanism of animals. Walter B. Cannon and Albert Moser were successful in their attempts, gradually developing a radiographic method of following ingested doses of opaque bismuth subnitrate as they traveled downward into the stomachs of cats. In July 1898, the two young men published their findings in a landmark paper in the *American Journal of Physiology*. That report has since become widely recognized as the first step toward establishing the field of gastrointestinal imaging. Their procedure fathered a host of progeny, including such common diagnostic methods as the GI series and the barium enema. Moser would die young, but Cannon went on to a distinguished career as a physiologist.

Max Nitze of the Allgemeines Krankenhaus, the Vienna General Hospital, had in 1879 added internal illumination and a new form of lens system to the rigid metal tubes with which unsatisfactory attempts were being made to look directly into the upper and lowermost parts of the digestive tract. His innovations were followed by rapid progress in the development of instruments to visualize not only the gut but the urinary and respiratory systems as well. By the turn of the century, the ground had been broken by the two techniques of radiology and direct visualization for major research and diagnostic studies of the esophagus, stomach, and bowel.

In the same year that the two young men from Harvard reported their success with the use of X rays, the thirty-nine-year-old director of the Institute for Experimental Medicine at St. Petersburg published in his native Russian a volume of 220 pages, *The Work of the Digestive*

Glands, that is universally acknowledged to be one of the most significant books in the long history of science. It is also the most important
contribution ever made to the understanding of the physiology of digestion. In elucidating the role of the central nervous system, and
later of the conditioned reflex, Ivan Petrovich Pavlov explored territories previously barely touched by his few predecessors in such work.
His studies of the gastric and intestinal secretions were revelatory.
They showed that psychological factors are of major significance; the
vagus nerve, originating in the medulla of the brain stem, is responsible for the connection between thoughts and digestion; different
kinds of foods produce different patterns of secretion; the percentage
of acidity of the gastric juice is constant; the secretion of gastric juice
is determined by chemical stimulation of the various glands that are
involved and not by the mechanical presence of food in the stomach;
there are three phases of gastric secretion, controlled by the nervous
system, the stomach, and the intestine, respectively.

Pavlov's enormous step represented the turning of a major corner
onto a route that would lead directly toward those extraordinary biomedical advances in the understanding of the digestive system that we
in the second half of the twentieth century have witnessed. The rapid
progress of recent decades has been made in a spirit of detached in-
quiry said by its exponents to be free of any subjective influence, and
certainly without resort to the long-abandoned habit of mystical
thought that in past centuries had been such a significant factor in the
interpretation of observed phenomena.

If the scientists' claim is justified and true, the rejection of any but
rational considerations must be seen for what it is—a conscious resistance against the straining forces within the human mind that turn in-
stinctively toward mysticism when reason has no ready explanation for
the mysteries still remaining in our biology. In attempting to explore
nature, we too readily succumb to the obsessional streak in ourselves
that seeks out with little provocation a way of elucidating based on ineffable powers we cannot know. Though we struggle mightily in its
grip, we will never conquer it. Science attempts to overcome the tendency to slip into the mystical, but must also recognize its constant

looming presence. Mankind naturally inclines in the opposite direction from critical thought; supernature and superstition supersede reason—reason is a hard-earned product of advanced civilization, requiring, like freedom, eternal vigilance lest the easier and more traditional ways engulf it.

CHAPTER FOUR

THE LIVER:

DUMB LUCK

AND THE SURGEON

W HEN Louis Pasteur uttered his now-famous aphorism, "Chance favors only the prepared mind," he was speaking of fortuitous occurrences that are experienced from time to time, which might be inconsequential or meaningless to most of us and yet present a great opportunity to the rare individual capable of recognizing their potential value. His little lesson is clear: Though anyone may stumble on an unanticipated scenario, only a few will know how to profit from it. An off-duty detective happening upon a crime will see things obscure or invisible to others who are present. A specialized researcher taking a casual peek down the barrel of someone else's microscope may discover wonders in a minuscule cellular landscape that is terra incognita to his colleague. By training, by experience, by skill, by a constant state of largely unconscious preparedness, some observers of a particular scene are able to make the most of whatever might unexpectedly present itself.

Surgery is a case in point. The underlying purpose of the years of a surgeon's rigorous training is the development of more than mere manual and cerebral dexterity—it is to reach a state of readiness that will allow the immediate interpretation of unfamiliar findings, an ability to take advantage of unforeseen opportunities, and the judgment to make appropriate decisions under urgent conditions. In prepared hands, chance can lead to cure. Or its proper use may save the day when danger looms.

The vast majority of situations in which a surgeon finds himself are governed by ground rules made familiar to him during the long period of training. Though the assorted variations and minefields I have described in the first chapter of this book add to the challenge and fascination of his daily doings, they rarely—very, very rarely—present an experienced operator with a problem he is unequipped to handle. Every once in a great while, he may deem it prudent to seek advice from a colleague, but such ad hoc consultations are usually intended more to reassure him that the path about to be taken makes good sense to an objective outsider than to direct him in his efforts.

None of this should be construed to mean that highly qualified surgeons never make mistakes, whether in technique or judgment. And it certainly should not be interpreted as assurance that those aforementioned exquisitely rare situations that are beyond a particular operator's—or sometimes *any* operator's—abilities are never encountered. An operation is an undertaking carried out by human beings on human beings—anything can happen.

Interwoven with all of the preceding is an unspoken factor that may occasionally determine the outcome of a surgical procedure. I call the factor "unspoken" because it never finds its way into the learned discussions at clinical conferences, or onto the pages of professional journals and books. I refer to the element we call luck. Being a profound believer in luck, I have more than once ruminated on why it may be good in one situation and bad in another; why some of us are more prone to its effects than are most; why an occasional person may with real justification be called lucky, while others seem dogged by the opposite so frequently that a mess is made of their lives, or at least their careers.

Kitchen-table philosophers are fond of the sententious "We make our own luck," and to a great extent they are right. By numerous qualities of personality and unconscious motivation—and yes, by the kind of deliberate preparedness described in the preceding paragraphs—factors within us can, not infrequently, determine the way in which unforeseen circumstances will play themselves out. It was specifically this to which Pasteur referred. And yet, not only lives but the course of major historical events as well have sometimes been known to turn on the fickleness of transient influences over which we have not an iota of control. Each of us has more than once found ourselves facing some unpredicted situation that could only have arisen from a figurative roll of the dice. Its outcome may be unrelated to anything we deliberately do.

For these reasons, I am a great believer in the effect of happenstance, the intangible ingredient that pops up in our lives when we least expect it. On a few occasions in my life, I have been extricated from a difficult situation not just by luck but by the indescribable form of it known as *dumb* luck.

Dumb luck has about it an element of being undeserved: a bad or good thing happens, perhaps in spite of us rather than because of us. In earlier times, the credit for happy outcomes was often given to such guiding factors as amulets and lucky stars, regardless of whether or not the grateful beneficiary believed in a Supreme Being. The religious who are untouched by superstition attribute their good fortune to God's intervention. Upon being safely delivered from peril or sickness, for example, an observant Jew recites a special prayer in which he says, "Blessed are You, Lord Our God, King of the universe, Who graciously bestows favor upon the undeserving, even as You have bestowed favor upon me." The implication is of having been granted unearned redemption.

Not only for unbelievers but also for those many people of faith who remain unpersuaded that God intervenes at every minor crossroads in our lives, there is luck to think about—that indeterminate, seemingly undetermined circumstance that makes things go one way or another, quite without contribution by the subject of it all. For such people, certain things just happen without reason—good or bad, deservedly or not.

Dumb luck has pulled my surgical chestnuts out of the fire on a few occasions when I felt certain that I was staring directly into the face of disaster. Whatever my preparedness may have contributed to the redemption of my patient and me at those times, it is difficult to believe that dumb luck did not weight to one side the balance in which we both sat, in a sense clasped in each other's arms. One of those occasions involved the liver.

THE events about to be related took place early in my career as a practicing surgeon in New Haven. Upon completing my training in 1961, I had spent a year in New York, most of which was devoted to setting up an open-heart surgery program at a six hundred–bed community hospital. Although the operations to be done were hardly new by then, there was undeniable risk in bringing them to an untried team in an institution unused to procedures of such magnitude. After the hospital's surgical chairman and I had successfully operated on our first few patients, I returned to New Haven secure in the belief that after such a challenge, there was little I might encounter in an OR that could intimidate me.

My story takes place a long time before the advent of trauma teams, paramedics, or personnel units dedicated solely to the treatment of emergencies. The ER duties in those days were handled by interns from the three clinical specialties of pediatrics, surgery, and internal medicine, with supervision provided, as required, by residents two or three years senior to them in the training process. If the intern felt he needed advice, one of the residents would leave his work on a patient care division and come down to the emergency room to provide it. On the surgical service, this meant that any patient deemed by the intern to need an urgent operation would be evaluated by the resident, who would review the situation and perform the necessary procedure himself unless private care was requested. In the latter eventuality, a call would be placed to the attending surgeon whose name was listed in that day's on-call panel.

The entire story I'm about to tell unfolded during six hours of a drizzly February Sunday during my second year of practice. I was living with my wife and our sixteen-month-old daughter in a garden apartment in the blue-collar town of East Haven, about three miles and a long, heavily traveled bridge from the hospital. The apartment had been chosen not only for its low rent but also because its proximity to the hospital meant that I could pull into the emergency room parking lot within six minutes of starting up the engine of my second-hand Ford Falcon.

The memorable call came at about six o'clock on that dreary evening, just as I was beginning to think about supper. There were no beepers in 1964, and I was accustomed to the phone ringing directly at home. An ER nurse was on the other end of the line, informing me that she knew few details beyond being told to have me come to the hospital right away. The surgical intern and several residents, she said, had ordered an OR to be readied as soon as possible for the woman about whom they were having me called. The patient was a thirty-one-year-old mother of two, in deep shock following the collision of her car with a light pole on one of the exits from I-95 in the Connecticut shoreline town of Guilford. On arriving in the ER by ambulance, the nurse reported, the woman had no pulse. Her blood pressure of 80/60 dropped to zero shortly afterward. The pulse rate could only be monitored by listening to her racing heartbeat. She was being rapidly transfused with A+ blood, which was the correct type, but there had been no time to match it specifically to her own red cells. She was also receiving an intravenous infusion of dextran, a fluid that expands plasma volume. The nurse apologized for speaking very quickly, explaining that she had to return immediately to the team, where she was needed in the urgent preparations for surgery.

Eight minutes later, I was pulling back the curtain at the ER location where three or four grim-faced young physicians and a small cadre of nurses were working tensely but with impressive expeditiousness over my new and obviously imperiled patient. An intern was just placing the last stitch into a four-centimeter gash over her left eyebrow. Directing the entire remarkably efficient coordination of so many individual efforts was a resident well known to me, in his fourth year of training. In spite of the hubbub of sound, Dr. Albert Dibbins had not raised his voice above an even tone of self-assurance, issuing quietly terse directions now to an intern, now to a nurse, as he stepped from one position to another around the gurney on which lay the severely injured patient. Al Dibbins was a short, somewhat heavyset man whose stocky build and thinning crew-cut hair complemented an air of emotional maturity and competence in such a natural way that he had always seemed to me much older than his age, which was then twenty-eight. In his accustomed manner, he was moving step by step and deliberately, but with great purpose.

It took but one sweeping glance over that busy arena to confirm that Dibbins had already brought everything under control—control, that is, within the limits of what was possible under the circumstances in which he had found his patient, whom I'll call Harriet Dale. Although orderly and in its own way reasonably calm, the scene had about it an ominous air of unbridled danger. Mrs. Dale's clothes had been hastily half cut, half torn from her wounded body and allowed to fall to the floor. Some of the bits of fabric having been kicked away by the personnel working feverishly alongside her, irregular fragments and shreds littered the area underfoot. The patient's naked form was exposed in full view under the stark brightness of a large surgical spotlight focused harshly on her abdomen.

A wide but barely perceptible puffiness extended transversely across the top of that tightly distended belly, a clear indication that the car's steering wheel had caught Mrs. Dale just under the rib cage. She groaned every time her belly was touched, no matter where. The foot of the gurney had been raised to assist what little blood was left in her pelvis and legs in making its way back to her speedily sprinting heart, which by then was pumping with just enough strength to produce a systolic blood pressure of 60. One of the nurses was bent over the patient's struggling form, monitoring the chest with a stethoscope. It could not have been easy to keep track of the birdlike ticking of the heartbeat—the restlessly thrashing woman was taking quick and very shallow respirations, more like grunted gasps than breaths. Although still alive, she was already pallid with the alabaster whiteness of impending death.

And yet the desperately injured woman was wide awake and speaking coherently. Ignoring gentle attempts by a nurse to speak soft, calming words into the moving target that was her right ear, she kept calling out, repeating over and over, "I can't see, I can't see—I'm blind! What's wrong? Why can't I see anything?" Although I was just a bit reassured by the evidence that her mind was clear, the blindness was worrisome. It meant that in spite of the transfusions of dextran and unmatched blood being hand-pumped by a nurse at each side of her, there was not sufficient volume to maintain more than barely adequate brain circulation. I found myself wondering—but only for a moment—whether the most useful service being performed for her would in the long run prove to be the one taking place neither around the gurney nor amidst the expeditious preparations upstairs in the OR, but the one being undertaken about ten feet away from all the activity to which I was witness: Though no one had asked any questions about religious affiliation, a young priest stood there, eyes fixed intently on the pages of an open prayer book, his lips barely moving as he intoned the last rites of the Catholic Church.

At that moment, my presence was superfluous. Dibbins was in command. The control he had taken of the situation would be wrested from him only to the patient's disadvantage. In any event, his management could not have been improved upon no matter how forcefully I might have inserted myself into the orbit of bustling rescue surrounding him.

Although the word had come that the OR would be ready within a few minutes, it would have been dangerous to upset our patient's tenuous circulatory equilibrium by moving her there until we were sure she would be transferred to the operating table immediately on arrival. But I felt compelled to do something useful for this woman whose life I now knew had been entrusted to my care. I settled for a thing less useful than I might have liked, but necessary nevertheless and even in the grand tradition of the barber-surgeons of yore. Grabbing a disposable razor from a nearby shelf, I shaved Mrs. Dale's pubis clear of hair with a few swift passes of the blade. As I finished, the word came that we could proceed up to the OR.

Most of the team was able to crowd with the gurney into the rickety superannuated elevator that would carry us to the OR suite on the fourth floor. By then, our patient was no longer able to speak, and her level of consciousness was uncertain. On the way up, Dibbins and I discussed our plan.

The one diagnostic certainty was that Mrs. Dale was bleeding into her abdomen. This much was obvious from the physical examination and the nature of the injury. An x-ray plate had been inserted under her upper back as the team worked on her, but the film obtained in this portable way was of such poor technical quality that it told us next to nothing. Our patient was too unstable and too short of time to allow even the quickest of trips to the second-floor radiology suite, so we could only hope that our interpretation of the physical exam was correct—specifically that there was no internal injury to the organs of the chest.

With blunt trauma and evidence of upper abdominal injury, the most likely cause of Mrs. Dale's instability was a rupture of the spleen, an organ particularly prone to be damaged by an accident of the sort she had sustained. The fact that she had complained of left shoulder pain on arrival in the emergency room supported that probability since pain in the spleen is often referred to the shoulder. The volume and rapidity of the bleeding was somewhat more than was usually seen with such a problem, but a complete shattering of the spleen might account for it. We decided that we would open the abdomen through a long incision parallel to the left rib margin.

One of the interns had preceded us to the OR and now stood scrubbed and gloved as we rushed our patient from the elevator and down the long corridor leading to the opened double doors of operating room 3. We rolled her gurney before us into the wide expanse of the old-fashioned, overly large space, and then I dashed down the hall toward the locker room to change into greens. When I returned no more than a minute later, the anesthesia team had transferred Mrs. Dale to the operating table and was checking her intravenous lines to be sure they were secure and dependable. Dibbins and a junior resident, both of whom had been wearing their OR greens all day, had completed a fast scrub, been gowned and gloved by the waiting nurses, and were ready to begin. As I started my own abbreviated scrub, the intern sloshed an antiseptic solution on the abdomen and hurriedly applied the sterile toweling and drapes. I was entering the room, arms up and with water dripping off my elbows, when the anesthetist announced that he had not been able to obtain a blood pressure since the patient's arrival in the OR suite. The pulse was 150, but it could be felt—and faintly at that—only by pressing firmly on the large artery in the groin. As fast as I could, I thrust myself into the gown and gloves being held out for me by the circulating nurse and took my place at the left side of the table.

Then I did something I had never attempted before and have never done since. Though there had not yet been sufficient time to anesthetize Mrs. Dale, I asked the anesthesiologist whether I had his permission to go ahead and make the incision anyway. He did not hesitate: "If you think you have to, go ahead. But I have no idea whether she'll feel it. Don't yell at me if she moves when you start cutting."

Dibbins hunched himself forward over the right side of the table with a finely balanced clamp—called a hemostat—hovering in each palm, poised to snap up bleeding arteries and veins when I sped across them with long sweeps of the scalpel. The intern, standing down-table alongside me, clutched an absorbent cloth sponge in one hand while holding the suction nozzle lightly between the fingertips of the other. He well knew how important his role would be. Without his efforts to keep the field dry of the expected outpouring of blood, Dibbins would not be able to see the incised vessels he was to clamp, and it would be impossible for me to cut through the layers of the abdominal wall as quickly as I needed to.

Palm turned upward, I extended my right hand toward the scrub nurse, and she slapped a scalpel into it. In that archaic high-ceilinged room, where the only other sound at that instant was the subdued murmuring of the anesthesiologist and his assistant as they hurriedly prepared to induce sleep, the knife's flat metal handle hitting against the tautly stretched rubber of my glove cracked like the sharp report of a pistol. It was as though a starter's gun had been fired, to set off what all of us huddled around our patient's heavily draped form knew would surely be a race against time and death.

Overwrought and clichéd though it may sound in this era when such scenes are commonplace on video and film, what I have just described was nevertheless the atmosphere of those few tense and yet eagerly expectant moments. Willy-nilly, everyone in that room—patient, doctors, nurses, each one of us—had been plunged into participation in a sequence of events that were rapidly unfolding precisely as they have been portrayed in literature and film. The members of our hastily assembled team were bound together with an intensity unimaginable to those who have not lived through such an experience or one of the few that may be comparable to it. Not a single individual among us was unaware that we were actors in the high drama that on rare occasions demands even more than the best of every person who works in operating rooms. Though the threat of failure hung over that scene like an unacknowledged wraith, it never occurred to me that it would descend to envelop us. To those gathered together in the effort to save a life, the certainty of success must be unquestioned.

Surgeons have been accused of many character flaws, but timidity is not among them. I stretched my hand forward over my patient's abdomen, lay the sharp edge of the scalpel on the chalk-white skin at the highest point of the arch under her ribs, and applied the gentlest of pressure. With a single continuous gliding movement, I cut through skin and fatty tissue. There being no response from the patient, it seemed safe to assume she felt nothing. As the anesthesiologist began the induction of sleep, our surgical team went ahead. The scrub nurse fired a glistening steel hemostat, then another into each of Dibbins's palms as he sequentially clamped the vessels I laid open on my journey down to the next layers. The exquisite precision and economy of movement during such proceedings, the smooth darting in and out of hands, and the choreography of skilled fingers—cutting, clamping, suctioning, sponging, and passing the delicately balanced instruments on their way to an open vessel—have always seemed a spectacle of ensemblelike beauty when I have seen it being carried out by others, but at the time of orchestrating such an effort, the only thought in the mind of its director is how fast and with what accuracy the whole performance can be accomplished.

In what seemed an instant, we found ourselves down to the peritoneum, the filmy translucent sheet that forms the inner layer enveloping the abdominal cavity. The wound was by then lined on each gaping side with a row of hemostats, whose tips held closed the cut ends of the many divided arteries and veins. Dibbins now quickly tied off the vessels with fine silk ligatures as I unclamped and removed the glistening steel instruments one after the other. The threads projecting from the final throw of every knot were cut short by the intern. Though still a plebe, he did his work with such exactness that at its conclusion the fleshy raw mound of incised abdominal muscle on each side looked like a pouting field of deep red lushness, specked with dozens of tiny black dots. Because of a combination of Dibbins's dexterity and our patient's state of deep shock, the edges of the sterile drape's opening were barely tinged with spilt blood.

The peritoneum bulged with the pressure of the scarlet tide pushing against it from within the abdominal cavity. When its thin texture was incised, the blood spilled out onto the drapes and soaked the sleeves of our gowns. I reached blindly with my left hand into the depths of the overflowing red pool and drew the spleen upward from the dense folds that held it to the back wall of the abdominal cavity and lateral margin of the stomach. To my intense relief, the pulpy blue-gray organ came forward a few inches. The maneuver was less difficult than I had anticipated, thanks to an unusual degree of flexibility of nearby tissues. With the tip of my submerged right index finger, I felt for the back layer of peritoneum behind the spleen and punched a hole through it. Then I literally tore the organ loose from its connections, until it was sufficiently free to break through the surface of the deep bloody pool. As the lacerated structure emerged into view, blood could be seen pouring out of a deep tear near the entry of its major arteries and veins. The flood stopped when Dibbins locked the parallel jaws of two clamps across the large vessels. The scrub nurse slapped a dissecting scissors into my hand, and I cut between the clamps, dividing the vessels and allowing the bulky specimen to drop into the kidney-shaped pan she held ready for it. A few heavy sutures were now placed individually into each of the vessels, and our job would seem to be done.

Not so. To our alarm, blood continued to pour in torrents from the opposite side of the abdomen, originating in a place we could not see.

With what sounded in that hushed room like one voice, Dibbins and I simultaneously barked, "It's the liver!" The words burst out with the stunned dismay that comes from the sudden realization of having missed something crucial that should have been obvious. It was as though a startlingly brutal light had just illumined the abyss of our joint stupidity. I muttered a few words to the scrub nurse and she slammed the scalpel into Dibbins's hand so that he might extend the incision along the opposite rib margin, directly over the liver's lower edge. I threw a series of clamps onto the bleeding vessels he cut through in the abdominal muscle, just as he had done previously, but this time we wasted no time tying them off. They were left to lie there as we quickly exchanged sides of the table, so that I was now on the right.

Blood was flooding out of a deep gash in the liver's central core, at a rate now so rapid that I feared a cardiac arrest might ensue if it could not be stopped within the next few seconds. I had never seen any complex liver surgery (with good reason: I later found out that none had ever been done at my hospital), and I had no idea what to do next. The acquired instantaneous responsiveness of long years of training—and certainly not deliberate thought—made me plunge my left hand blindly through the blood toward a thick curtain of tissue just below the organ's huge rubbery bulk and wrap my fingers tightly around it. The fat-enveloped fold I now grasped was a structure called the porta hepatis, or gateway to the liver, known by this designation since Galen gave it that name, at a time when the liver was called the hepar.

The porta, as it is familiarly known, holds three major structures within a surrounding covering of fatty tissue: the duct carrying bile downward from liver to intestine; the common hepatic artery, supplying the liver; and the portal vein, a short, wide channel that transports into the liver all blood returning from the spleen and virtually the entire length of the digestive tract. Although I had never seen it done, my snug encirclement of the porta constituted what has long been called the Pringle maneuver, whose purpose is to gain control over the liver's blood supply. I clung to the garroted mass of tissue as though to dear life, which is precisely the precarious situation into which Mrs. Dale had been thrust.

To explain what now presented itself to our worried inspection, it is necessary to say a few words about the anatomy of the liver, which at some 1200 grams (about 2½ pounds) in weight is by far the heaviest and largest of the solid structures in the body, except, of course, for the brain.

Although the liver looks like a single unit, it is in fact made up of a left and a right lobe, each served by one of the two divisions into which

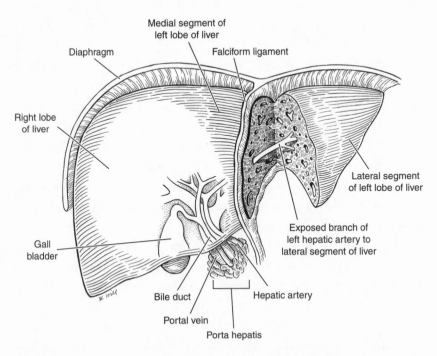

Diagram of the injury to Harriet Dale's liver. The injury is depicted as being deeper than it actually was, in order to demonstrate the appearance of the lacerated surfaces.

the bile duct, the hepatic artery, and the portal vein, respectively, are separated. The left lobe is further divided into a medial (adjacent to the right lobe) and a lateral segment, their junction identifiable on the organ's surface by a front-to-back groove running along the plane that separates them. A strong, thin sheet of fibrous tissue is attached to the top of the liver along this groove, and its upper edge merges into the diaphragm above and the abdominal wall in front. This sheet, called the falciform ligament, serves to anchor the liver to both of these sturdy structures. Obviously, it also serves as a useful external guide to recognizing the plane of demarcation between the medial and lateral segments.

What Dibbins and I were looking at with such disquiet was a deep fracture extending halfway through the structure of the left lobe of the liver, along the falciform ligament. It was as though someone had chopped with an axe into the furrow between medial and lateral segments, and then spread them apart as much as was allowed by the bridge of remaining uncut tissue deep within the injury. The liver lay before us like an opened book of ten chapters, spread widely at the end of chapter 7. The separated segments gaped, held together by the intact liver only across the back of the organ, as though it was the book's binding. As long as I kept squeezing on the porta hepatis, blood oozed only from the raw surfaces of the spread-apart tissue, mixed with a profuse flow of bile. But when I let loose for a moment, a torrential outpouring came forth, obscuring the operative field and worrying the hell out of me.

At the best of times, the liver is a difficult organ to work with, having the consistency of spongy gelatin and holding stitches poorly. Attempts to burn the bleeding surface with electric cautery are usually to no avail. Still, the injuries I had encountered in previous patients had been well controlled with large, strategically placed sutures, but only because these wounds had been much less extensive than the one presented by Mrs. Dale. The few patients with more complicated hepatic trauma who survived to reach a hospital in those days were customarily treated by tightly packing the lacerated organ with large sponges and a coagulant material called Gelfoam. The abdomen would then be reexplored after some days, when sufficient strengthening of clot was thought to have taken place to permit the removal of the packing. The danger of infection and late hemorrhage made such methods hazardous, and they were only used in desperation. Even had I wanted to employ this technique, though, it was probable that no amount of packing would suffice to stanch this deeply wounded liver.

Faced with the impossibility of repairing the enormous hepatic injury with sutures, and the minimal likelihood that packing would succeed, I was promptly engulfed by unaccustomed pessimism. There seemed no way to proceed. Though our patient was still alive—with blood pressure and pulse responding, in fact, to the blood being pumped into her—I felt myself without options. I could think of no way to save the young woman whose life was in my frustrated hands. But Dibbins had no doubts. "Let's take it out," he said, and for an instant I thought he had lost his senses under the pressure of those terrible moments. "It's being done in some places, so why not?"

A few large clinical centers at which certain of the faculty were highly experienced in the treatment of trauma had indeed begun to recommend the resection, or excision, of entire lobes or segments when liver injuries were very difficult to treat otherwise. Surgeons were still so unfamiliar with inner hepatic anatomy, however, that authors of the scant number of published articles would make a point of including in their publications detailed diagrams of the techniques they were in the process of developing. But even in that tiny vanguard of institutions, the number of patients was still small, and the method had hardly caught on. At the vast majority of American hospitals, emergency major liver resections had not yet been attempted. In the previous year, in fact, one of the largest teaching centers in the United States had published an article describing a series of 111 patients with liver injuries of all kinds, not one of whom had undergone a resection. On that Sunday afternoon so many years ago, it was doubtful that many American surgeons had any idea of how to go about doing complex hepatic operations.

Neither Dibbins nor I, for example, was able to name the intact artery we saw, curving like a miniature pipe across the gap between the two partially separated pieces of the lobe. We did recognize a wide-open segment of vessel as being a torn bit of the left portal vein. Beyond this and identifying one large and many small openings leaking amber secretions from the peripheral tributaries of the bile duct, we knew only that we were in a dreadful jam. Neither of us had so carefully studied the isolated reports of hepatic resection that we were familiar with their abstruse details. In fact, we did not even appreciate that the left lobe has two segments. The answer to Dibbins's "Why not?" was that we did not know how.

He had made an audacious suggestion. To implement it, I would have to make up the operation as I went along. This would necessitate cutting or tearing my way by dead reckoning through the remaining still-intact liver behind the laceration as it poured out blood and bile. I would have to do this while sequentially stitching the profusion of small ducts and vessels as they appeared, even though we could not identify them by name. But first, it would be necessary to place individual sutures into the many conduits that were now emptying their yellow and red contents onto the operative field. Since hepatic tissue is too fragile to hold stitches, I would have to guide my needle with perfect accuracy into the relatively sturdy walls of the conduits themselves. Hours of painstaking work would be required, and even if I successfully accomplished it, there was no certainty of the stitches holding or that the vast surface of raw liver would heal without infection or delayed hemorrhage.

Who knows what I might have done without Dibbins's suggestion. Left to my own devices, it is not unlikely that I would have resorted to the time-honored if rarely effectual method of tight and hopeful packing. Had I done so, it would almost certainly have cost my patient her life, but seeking refuge in a familiar technique would evoke little criticism from my peers. A death following the orthodox treatment of so extensive an injury is acceptable to a surgeon's conscience. Moreover, such an outcome would have been far more justifiable to my colleagues at our weekly complications conference than would a mortality resulting from a hastily conceived attempt at an operation I had never seen and was hardly familiar with.

These were the thoughts that were racing through my disquieted mind as I wasted precious seconds trying to decide what to do. Should I rely on the easily defensible standard and thereby virtually ensure my patient's death, or should I take the radical route that might save her and risk the condemnation of my fellow surgeons if it did not succeed? It took only a few more moments to realize that Dibbins had presented me with the only possible strategy. It was clear that this was Mrs. Dale's one realistic chance for survival. I decided to take a perilous flight by the seat of my pants, but in fact I had no choice. It was this or almost certain failure.

Having made the decision, I briefly discussed tactics with the team. It was clear that the force of the blunt trauma had torn the liver along a plane continuous with the falciform ligament, the ligament's attachment having served as a fixed line on which the shearing force had exerted itself. It seemed to make sense that the best way to complete the division of the remaining liver tissue was to continue along that plane. At this point, ignorance of the anatomy precluded our knowing something that we would realize only later: The injury had occurred precisely along the boundary between the left lobe's medial and lateral segments. This meant that we were unknowingly about to complete an operation beginning to be referred to in the very small number of surgical papers on the subject as a lateral segmentectomy of the left hepatic lobe. We would be cutting through the figurative open book's binding and discarding the final three chapters.

But first, all of the tubular structures lying open on the wide expanse of the "final page of chapter 7" needed to be stitched. I began by guiding the intern's hand to the porta hepatis to replace mine. Being in the boundary zone between medial and lateral segments (although we did not know it), the injured tributary of the portal vein had been torn tangentially, so that about a half inch of it lay open as if a piece of its wall had been cut away. In spite of the intern's tight hold on the porta, the vein had continued to ooze dark blood, making it difficult to see its torn edges as I began to run a hair-thin silk suture over and over along its jagged rim. I was careful to place the delicate curved needle only into the sturdy wall of the vein, avoiding as much as possible the undependable mushiness of the injured liver tissue around it. Dibbins helped by holding the suction tip directly over the site to aspirate away the seeping blood that obscured my line of sight as I worked. But even with the visibility improved that way, it took longer than I would have liked before I had completed placing the length of the stitch and tied it down. To my immense relief, it held securely. The large vessel was no longer bleeding.

Except for a gaping hole, the yellowish color of whose slow, sticky leakage revealed that it was the open end of the left branch of the bile duct, the largest tubular structure in sight was the pulsating bit of miraculously undamaged artery curving across the open space between the two parts of the liver (from the last page of chapter 7, as it were, across to the first of chapter 8), that my assistants and I were still unable to identify. Dibbins now clamped the vessel's midpoint with the tips of two parallel hemostats. I cut between them and he stitched the ends closed. After a suture was next placed in the gaping bile duct, we turned our attention to the wide, raw surface of the main part of the liver, which would remain in the patient.

One by one, we stitched each of the open channels on the oozing tissue's broad expanse. To lessen blood loss, the work on the vessels was done first, before we turned our attention to the bile ducts. Every few minutes, the intern was instructed to relax his hold on the porta hepatis for several seconds, to "give the liver a drink." Hepatic cells are very sensitive to oxygen deprivation; even though the field was briefly flooded with bright-red blood each time he let go, frequent nourishment of the liver was critical to keeping it alive. Working meticulously, we took more than two hours to complete the demanding job of closing every one of the dozens of tubular structures, but at the end we were able to gaze with satisfaction on the wide expanse of surface to the right of the cleavage plane. Although the tissue was still just a bit wet, not a single duct or vessel of any size remained open.

The next task was to determine how best to complete the dissection begun by Mrs. Dale's steering wheel. The gaping gash extended about halfway through the liver, and the "book's binding" would have to be divided. To cut directly through it with a scalpel or even an electric cautery would have resulted in yet another outburst of rapid bleeding.

Even worse, the ends of some of the freshly divided vessels might pull back or retract into the hepatic tissue and be impossible to clamp. The best approach, I decided, was to push through it with the blunt handle of the scalpel. Since the larger conduits had sturdy walls of elastic consistency, my hope was that I could find them simply by pushing away their surrounding liver tissue. Once exposed, they could be stitched before being injured.

Using my scalpel in this way, and also by pinching hepatic substance between the tips of my index finger and thumb, I was able to do as I intended. It was not until I consulted my surgical journals the next day that I discovered my impromptu stratagem to be the technique advised by the author who had had the most experience with such operations. It was also while reading his article that I found the name of the intact vessel crossing the field: lo and behold, it was the main artery to the lateral segment of the left lobe. The steering wheel had exposed it lying there in the plane between the medial and lateral lobes, just as I would have done had I planned the dissection. But of course, to plan the dissection, I would have had to know what I was doing.

Placing stitches into the channels before actually cutting across them avoided all but minimal further blood loss. When I had pinched through the last bit of liver, Dibbins lifted the excised specimen out of the abdomen and briefly held it up for everyone to see. He then carefully lowered it into the waiting hands of the scrub nurse. She dropped it into the pan and wagged an index finger at it. "Naughty, naughty," she scolded. "Look at all the trouble you caused." She had put into words what every member of our very relieved team was surely thinking.

The tiniest divisions of the blood and bile passages are not only too small to stitch but they are not even identifiable to the naked eye. Though we had sewn up every open channel that could be seen, the raw liver surface—the "final page of chapter 7"—would predictably ooze, albeit very slowly, until it was covered over with clot and, later, scar. It seemed clear that the best way to minimize postoperative leak would be to attempt to close the open tissue with a series of stitches.

The liver is enveloped in a thin but quite strong envelope of transparent fibrous material called Glisson's capsule. I placed a row of

stitches intended to snug the front, or anterior, edge of the cut capsule to the back, or posterior, edge—thereby closing the liver like a
purse. I did this by laying a row of individual catgut sutures into position, each one picking up a generous bit of capsule in front and then
in back. When I pulled up on the stitches and tied them firmly down,
I found that the two edges did come together quite nicely. Just to provide some layers of insurance, I cut loose the edge of falciform ligament from the front of the abdominal wall and stitched it down over
the line of sutures, and then added a flap of peritoneum from the
back of the abdominal cavity. In carrying out these maneuvers I was
once more unaware that I was following the published suggestion of
an expert. When I got through with everything, it looked as though
nature herself had done the job. After positioning two suction tubes
under the operative area to aspirate any fluid that might drain out in
spite of all precautions, we closed the abdomen with a layer of strong
silk sutures to the peritoneum and braided wire to the muscle and
fibrous tissue. Mrs. Dale was then brought out of the anesthesia as
easily as though she had just undergone a standard sixty-minute
operation on her gallbladder.

Dibbins and I were pleased with ourselves, but we were hardly at the
end of our worries: Our patient would not be free of the threat of bile
leak, bleeding, or infection for weeks. Though we believed she would
do perfectly well with almost a third of her liver in a laboratory jar, we
were not absolutely sure. Our uncertainty extended to the possibility
that some other injury might lie deep within the remaining liver,
which we had no way of identifying because it had presented no external manifestations. The massive hemorrhage and the physiological
insult of the prolonged period of shock as well as the trauma of such
an extensive operation might give rise to as yet unforeseen postoperative problems.

Still, it was difficult to resist the powerful euphoria that overcame
the entire team as we contemplated what we had just done. No matter
what might happen in the next few days, there was no way we could be
deprived of our technical accomplishment, which at that moment
overshadowed in our minds even the fact that a young wife and
mother had been snatched back from the verge of death. Under un-

remitting pressure, Dibbins and I had improvised an enormously demanding operation and carried out its minutest details with such perfection as to represent, as we saw it, the epitome of the surgeon's art. We were button-busting proud of ourselves.

As the breathing tube was being removed from the awakening woman's windpipe, the circulating nurse informed me that my patient's husband was waiting in the lobby. He had arrived at the hospital shortly after Mrs. Dale was rushed to the OR. Because of the feverish fluster with which we had begun operating and then the intensity of the procedure itself, no one had remembered to transmit any information to him. All he knew was how perilously sick his wife had been when she was wheeled from the emergency room. His last bit of information had come when one of the interns phoned him five hours earlier to obtain his permission for operation. In our haste and concern for the problem before us, not a single member of our very young team had thought to send word to him about his wife's condition.

I stripped off gown and gloves. Without thinking to change out of my blood-caked greens, I got myself back into the same rickety elevator that had brought us all to the OR. I pulled its clumsy gate shut with the clanging slam of renewed energy and rode down to the first floor. It was eleven-thirty at night, and there was no one in the corridor as I walked briskly, with the enthusiasm of triumph, toward the information desk. As I entered the empty lobby I saw a tall, stooped figure pacing a short path back and forth alongside one of the overstuffed chairs that are the standard furniture of such places. He dropped his lean frame into it just as I came up behind him, and slumped dejectedly into its depths. I was too full of myself to think about the torment he had been suffering.

Even now, several decades later, I am almost too ashamed to tell what I did next. I stepped in front of Mr. Dale, thrust my arm forward, and pumped his limp, unresponsive hand, while he looked up at me stunned, as though a bloody apparition had appeared to confirm his worst fears. "Mr. Dale, I'm Dr. Nuland, and I've just operated on your wife. The steering wheel slammed into her liver, so we had to take out a large piece of it. It's a very rare operation, but I'm really pleased that we were able to pull it off. The whole team was great—just great." I must have sounded like the charged-up captain of a basketball team that had just won the national championship.

Peter Dale blinked two or three times, very slowly, as the ebullient words burst out of me at machine-gun speed. He seemed not to care, or perhaps he was uncomprehending of what I was telling him. Until he spoke, I had no realization of the magnitude of my indifference to his distress. His words and the sudden sharpness of their tone belied the passivity of what was, up to that instant, his slouched, defeated mien. In the flash of an eye blink, he went from seeming lethargy to a manner at once irritated and impatient—and then pleading.

"I don't care about any of that," he snapped. And more slowly, "Just tell me how my wife is. Please just tell me—is she going to live?" I was jerked back into the reality of the near-tragedy I had been neglecting because of my vainglorious absorption with the technical feat of having resected a big hunk of liver under such challenging circumstances—my absorption, in fact, with myself.

I was mortified. Not only the man's words but the sudden awareness of how I must seem to him—the archetypal self-worshiping surgeon, concerned only with his technology, his team, and himself—filled me with a profound sense of humiliation, even a loathing of what I must appear in his eyes to be. The puffed-up pride of accomplishment had no place here. For almost five hours this desperate man had been waiting alone, in the deepest anxiety, for a few words of comfort, and I had given him an uncaring display of egotism.

I looked down toward my feet and mumbled an apology. And then, "Yes, yes, she's fine. She's waking up from the anesthesia and you'll have her home in about two weeks, good as new." I was saying more than I felt sure about, but at that instant I owed this man something very big. It was not enough to have given him back his wife—I had to make up for the way I had told him about it. An excess of optimism seemed just right, exactly what was called for.

He smiled at me—a large, sweet, and suddenly very warm smile. He stood up, towering three skinny inches over me, his droopy red-brown mustache stretched across his upper lip by the sheer width of that beaming grin. This time it was *he* who pumped *my* hand. I could feel something choking up in my throat, and I knew that my eyes glistened with just the beginning of the emotion I could now allow myself, of contrition and pleasure both. "I'm sorry," I said again. "I'm sorry for how I told you. It's just that . . ." I heard my voice trail off, as I realized I was all at once feeling like a child in need of forgiveness, and approval too. He must have sensed it. "It's OK," he replied. "As long as I know she's all right."

Harriet Dale proved to be better than just all right. Although she did have a brief episode of pneumonia (almost certainly caused by aspiration of stomach contents during the unorthodox induction of anesthesia), it cleared up rapidly, and the rest of her course was smooth thereafter. She went home even before the two weeks were up. It was obvious from the first postoperative day that she was a woman of keen intelligence and a wry sense of humor, a woman who kept all of us off balance by her perceptive—and sometimes acid—observations of hospital life and every member of the treatment team.

And she did something else for us as well. Because of reports of regeneration of liver in experimental animals (and a startling article from Memorial Sloan-Kettering Cancer Center describing the same thing in four patients, published only months earlier), I ordered a sequence of radionuclide scans to evaluate this possibility. On the third study, six months after operation, almost all of the absent tissue had reappeared, growing leftward like a budding yeast from the cut surface of the organ. By this time, Mrs. Dale was fed up with being seen as a patient. Moreover, she was concerned about the possible long-term effects of the radiation, "done only to satisfy your surgical curiosity," and no amount of reassurance or coaxing would change her determined mind. That ended the studies but not the follow-up. As recently as 1997, we met again when I visited Seattle, where she now lives. She has never had a bit of trouble related to the formidable operation done on that drizzly Sunday evening way back in 1964, when we were both a great deal younger.

I introduced the story of Harriet Dale by calling it an occasion on which I and a patient were saved by dumb luck. I might well be asked at this point, "What about the role of those qualities you described on the first page of this chapter as so often being decisive at moments when chance shows its face—training, skill, experience, and a constant state of unconscious preparedness?" Certainly the operation could not have succeeded had those elements been absent. They allowed me, à la Pasteur, to make the most of the situation that arose. But without some dumb luck, I argue, nothing would have availed.

First, there was the presence of Al Dibbins. Any one of six residents at his level of training might have chanced to be on duty that weekend. Looking back on their respective states of resourcefulness—and daring, as well—it is extremely unlikely that any of the other five would have made the suggestion that Dibbins did. Would I have thought of it on my own? Assuming that I did—which was far from having been a certainty—was his obvious enthusiasm a factor in my decision to go ahead with it? Did his presence serve as a goad, or perhaps a reassurance? I'll never know, and that's fine with me.

But the master stroke of dumb luck involved not a scintilla of human intervention—it was a simple fact of physics and anatomy: The steering wheel had hit Harriet Dale's abdomen at such an angle and transmitted such a shearing force that it caused a tear along exactly the plane of demarcation between the medial and lateral segments of the liver's left lobe. Had I deliberately set out to resect the lateral segment, studied the anatomy and the suggested technique with diligence, and followed the directions with scrupulous care, I would have found myself beginning the operation by doing precisely what the steering wheel accomplished when it sheared off the front half of the organ. The injury had gone so far as to expose the curving arch of the left hepatic artery as it entered the segment, leaving it lying intact and cleanly exposed there, just waiting to have hemostats clamped across it—as though a spirit-surgeon had dissected it out for me. A bit more force and the artery would have been severed, adding just enough hemorrhage to kill its victim within minutes of injury; a bit less and I might have torn into it inadvertently while making my way through the remaining liver tissue. By laying out the plan of dissection and carrying it up to a point but not beyond, Harriet Dale's dumb luck—and therefore mine—had not only done half my work for me but provided a road map for the rest. Without the guidance of luck, I might have become irretrievably lost in the complex network of vessels and ducts within the liver's substance, and been unable to extricate myself and my patient. Sometimes an inanimate object—even a steering wheel—is the best assistant.

And sometimes too, Professor Pasteur, we need more than just a prepared mind.

CHAPTER FIVE

THE LIVER:

SOURCE OF LIFE

Is it possible to imagine an organ regenerating a lost part of itself, without being struck by a sense of wonder that such a thing can actually happen? Musings on that reality must surely be first cousin to the fantasy of resurrection of the body itself, and of eternal life. Though the injured liver's ability to accomplish its marvel was first observed in dogs only as recently as 1890, legends of magical regenerations—and even a transplant or two—seem always to have adorned the lore of many cultures, a close relative to the belief in reincarnation. Humankind's inability to face the finality of death has twisted itself into protean forms, all meant to deny the permanence of that ultimate snuffing out of consciousness, beyond which we exist only in the history of what we were.

Myths of regeneration, with their implied promise of a renewal of life, accorded well with primitive man's simplest observations of nature. Flora seem to die each autumn, and yet they do not. Some animals are not seen for months, only to reappear in the spring. The seasons, the tides, the settings and risings of the sun—the ebbing and flowing of all he knows—reassure *Homo sapiens* of the cycles that restore life when the proper time has come.

And so it must have been also, with the healing of wounds and recovery from disease. Nowadays we are so quick to intervene with treatment at the earliest evidence of sickness that we incline to forget what our forebears knew well: The vast majority of indispositions—and not only the minor ones—are cured by the restorative powers of nature. A worsening course reverses itself, and vitality appears once more. A sick person arises from bed like a phoenix, prepared for yet another episode of life. The phoenix story, in fact, is a universal fantasy of wish-fulfillment.

Though the myth of the phoenix is associated with Egypt, its origins may be even more ancient, and attributable to an earlier culture in the Orient. After a life span of five hundred years, the fabled bird was said to light a fire to its nest, in whose flames it was itself consumed. Arising from its own ashes, the brilliantly plumed creature lived again, to repeat the process twice in each millennium. So deeply implanted has it always been in the fantasy of man's mind that the theme of death and resurrection has defied all attempts to identify its historic roots. They will never be found. Tales of floods and phoenix-fires, redemption and renewal, sin and purification precede even early religions. They exist because we need them.

Such legends abound in both pagan and modern belief systems. Whether with the sincere conviction of the born-again Christian or the pop psychology of such verbal nostra as "Today is the first day of the rest of your life," we seek renewal and thrive on its promise. Many pocket editions exist of the coming of the Messiah, portable and ready for daily use. There seems never to have been a time when we have not woven these themes into our storytelling. Even the Mesopotamian Gilgamesh epic of four thousand years ago, for example, was probably not the first account of floods and the search for renewed youth.

And so, when clear evidence was obtained that Harriet Dale had regenerated her lost liver, I could not help but muse over the symbolism of it all. Whether by dumb luck (as I believe) or Divine Providence (as some others might say), she had, in a sense, been raised from the dead. As a visible metaphor for her restored life, the left lateral lobe of her liver had grown back. It was impossible not to think of the Greek myth of Prometheus.

Prometheus—the word itself means "forethought," and the name is an integral part of his myth. Being endowed with forethought, Prometheus had qualities that enabled him to become the master craftsman, the creator of man. Proud of his accomplishment, he determined to bestow on his creation dominance over all other living creatures. But only if man possessed fire could this come to pass, and therein lay the rub. Fire was owned by the gods, and they would not willingly share it.

Prometheus's reputation as a great trickster had already angered Zeus, during an earlier episode when he fooled the chief god into accepting the fat and bones of a sacrificial bull in place of the animal's meat. When the mischief was compounded by the theft of fire to give to mortals, punishment was swift and terrible. Zeus seized Prometheus, chained him to a great rock, and sent a bloodthirsty vulture to feast on his liver.

All day long, the vicious bird would tear out pieces of his anguished victim's liver, but the devoured tissue would grow back again when night fell. In this way, the regeneration that should have meant new life resulted instead only in more agony, as the vulture returned again and again. Prometheus was tortured anew each day for many generations, until finally he was rescued by Heracles.

Mankind responded with gratitude and blessings to the benisons granted by Prometheus. Mythology credits him with being the inventor of medicine, astronomy, architecture, and writing; the gift of fire was, in effect, the gift of enlightenment—the gift of civilization itself. It was the factor that ensured much of mankind's uniqueness. The possession of fire would in time enable humans to learn the secrets not only of the gods above but of the earth below as well, and thereby to develop science, commerce, and the arts. No wonder that we use the adjective *Promethean* to mean "creative" and "life-giving."

The derivation of *Promethean* is characteristic of the way in which the evolution of language is a key to the early history of our culture, and so is the name of the organ being discussed. The word *liver* is described in Shipley's *Origins of English Words* as deriving from an Indo-European root, *leip,* that is associated with life, related to the ancient assumption that this structure is the seat of life—of living—because it was believed to manufacture the blood. In Middle English, spoken at the height of influence of the old Galenic doctrines, the word was *lifer.* Following the same pathway, the German is *die Leber,* in a language whose verb *to live* is *leben.* In the days when philology was a thriving academic pursuit, this sort of detective work brightened the hours of many a cloistered scholar.

With all of this as background, it hardly seems a coincidence that the mythological character who gave life and fire to mankind should be punished by having his liver chewed at by a ravenous vulture. Hidden as they are within the dense fabric of modern culture, the interweaving threads of a civilization's memory may be difficult to find, but they have not disintegrated.

Based on its presumed role as the maker and reservoir of the blood, the notion of the liver as the seat of life and perhaps the center of the soul is at least as old as the time of the great Mesopotamian city of Babylon that thrived some eighteen to twenty centuries B.C.E. It was the Mesopotamian custom to bring a live sheep to the temple for sacrifice before the statue of a god, particularly if a prediction about illness was sought. If the solicitant was too sick to be moved, he would breathe into the animal's nostrils prior to a surrogate's setting out with it. Once the sheep had been killed, its liver was removed and carefully inspected by a soothsayer of the temple, as was the cavity in which it had lain. The theory behind this was that the god's acceptance of the sacrifice meant that he identified with the spirit of the animal and therefore would make his intentions known through the organ that represented the soul.

This was no haphazard process. During his novitiate, the priest would have been trained in this form of divination, using a clay model of a sheep's liver marked up into numerous rectangles by a series of intersecting lines on its surface. Each of these many areas had a distinctive name and represented specific characteristics. Archeologists have found such models not only in Mesopotamia and surrounding lands but in Tuscany as well, indicating that the art of what historians call hepatoscopy was practiced in the Italian peninsula as late as the Etruscan period, during the sixth century B.C.E.

The divination had a consistent logic about it. Each anatomical variation of the sacrificed sheep's liver was noted by the soothsayer, whether of the organ itself or of its blood vessels and bile ducts. No observation, regardless of its magnitude or nature, was neglected. Everything was considered to have meaning, according to well-defined criteria that had been recorded in scripture. Should any of the squares contain or lie over an abnormality, no matter how minor, this fact was interpreted to reveal some portent. Thus, even a small hepatic surface marking or bit of an outgrowth would have great significance, as obviously would a tumor or evidence of infection. Liver disease being common among sheep at the time, various manifestations of infection added wide variety to the observations that could be made. Even the normal liver has so many anatomical variations that these, too, entered into the total prediction.

Although the priest did not cut into the liver, the divinations depended on more than surface evidence alone. The characteristics of the gallbladder, blood vessels, and ducts as well as the size and shape of the lobes were also factors. Depending on the totality of his findings, the priest made a prediction about the petitioner's health. But not only health was the purview of the soothsayer. His skills were employed as well to predict a wide range of future events and to give counsel when decisions were to be made. Thus, in the Book of Ezekiel (21:21) we find Nebuchadnezzar, the king of Babylon, apparently at a crossroads on his way to battle: "For the king of Babylon stood at the parting of the way, at the head of the two ways, to use divination: he made his arrows bright, he consulted with images, he looked in the liver."

Other references exist, in scripture and later sacred writings, of the ways in which the liver was thought by the ancients to be the center of life. In all ways, the centrality of the liver among certain civilizations was unquestioned, all because of its association with the blood. The soul is thus seen as a movable feast—at various times in history it was thought to reside in the liver, the stomach, the heart, and finally the brain. We seek it still.

(It should be pointed out that the words *soul, psyche* [*psuche,* in the original Greek], and the Latin *anima* are being used synonymously in this book. In general, there are minimal and frequently no differences among their usage by various authors of either earlier or present times.)

One of the archeological evidences of liver divination as practiced by the Etruscans is a bronze representation of a sheep's liver found in 1877 near the Tuscan city of Piacenza. It consists essentially of a five-inch plate from which several tuberosities protrude. Its surface bears the inscribed names of Etruscan gods. Spread out along the length of its edge is a series of sixteen marked divisions, each with a region of the cosmos named on it. Because of the association of the liver with gods and heavenly bodies, it has been suggested that the bronze artifact represents the communion of microcosm and macrocosm in soothsaying.

This notion, too, seems to go back to Babylonian times. The Mesopotamians, like so many other peoples, believed that the biological cycle of the earth and of individuals was determined by the positions and movements of the heavenly bodies. The cycles they saw in the heavens seemed to them coordinated with the cycles they saw on earth, of fertility, maturation, death, and renewal. The predictability of these cycles must have been very reassuring to the ancient mind. In time it would all blend together into the generalized theory developed in Greece that both microcosm and macrocosm are composed of the four primary elements of earth, air, fire, and water, and the four qualities of heat, cold, moistness, and dryness, all related in turn to the humors, as described earlier. Like all other living things, humans are therefore at one with the universe. (Parenthetically, it hardly need be pointed out that the word *atone* literally means to return to a oneness—to be at one, a unity—a notion traceable to the earliest concepts of man's relation to the surrounding universe, and later to God.)

In such ways, man gradually came to place himself and his society within the influence of the cycles of the natural world, subject to and reassured by the same rhythms, consistencies, and renewals he saw everywhere around him. In a world made chaotic by the unpredictability of sprites, forest elves, and fanciful beings of all kinds, it must have been comforting to believe that humans are somehow a part of an ongoing, predictable totality. No matter the turbulence he may have sensed inside and around himself, early man needed to believe that there was an ultimate harmony to life. It was the harmony that cocooned him in its nurturing center; it was the harmony he sought to re-create in his society and the regularized patterns of his culture. The search for a source of harmony and a connection to the cosmos is in a direct way related to the notion of soul, a living factor transcending flesh and providing intimations of higher and immortal forces within and without.

In this connection, it is interesting to observe that Plato's notions of the soul are related to the liver. In his view, as expressed in *Timaeus*, "soul" is a three-part concept, embodying all the activities that give the body its organized functioning. Highest of the three is the divine psyche, an immortal source of rationality dwelling in the head and associated with the cosmic force that governs the universe. The emotional psyche, on the other hand, is housed in the chest, with the heart. The nutritive, or baser, psyche is in the abdomen. The role of the liver is to bring the stomach, spleen, and intestines under the rational control of the divine psyche. It is able to do this because it is smooth and shiny and therefore capable of reflecting images coming from that higher source. It supplements this ability with the capacity for bitterness and sweetness, so that it may respond to the influence of the highest psyche in such a way as to transmit those influences to its fellow abdominal organs.

It is worth noting that Plato does mention that the liver of a sacrificed animal can be used to interpret dreams. The continuity of his thought with the past is consistent with the continuity of his thought in so many other areas of philosophy. As moderns looking back on the millennia-old history of ideas, we are so absorbed with the original contributions of our intellectual forebears that we ignore—sometimes

to our disadvantage—that their ideas arose in the context of their cultural heritage. There are no purely *de novo* thinkers, or at least none
who make lasting contributions. In being creatures of our time, we are
creatures of all that has come before. Even the true believer in renewal, rebirth, and resurrection must deal with that little prefix, "re."

Until William Harvey would consign it to history by describing the
circulation, belief in the liver's centrality persisted in various forms.
But along the way, there were always a few naysayers. Among them was
Aristotle, who believed that the body's most important organ is the
heart. To him, it was not only the source of the blood and vital heat but
the seat of the soul as well.

After Galen encoded his notions of digestion and blood production
five hundred years after Aristotle, very few authorities had the temer-
ity to disagree with them. In the scheme of the great mahatma of medicine, two by-products were left when the liver made blood: the thick
and dark black bile that was stored in the spleen; and the thin and
light yellow bile that left the liver with the blood. It was Galen's contention that the liver housed a natural spirit to direct the whole
process, not only of nutrition but also of the ebbing and flowing by
which, he asserted, blood reached the periphery of the body. Once
there, he taught, the tissues took from the blood according to their
needs. Although Galen did believe that the heart is the prime source
of the body's innate heat, he wrote that the liver, too, makes a contribution.

Like so many of his predecessors, Galen asserted that the liver is the
source of life. The evidence, he claimed, was to be found in its embryonic development. Noting that the organ is proportionally larger in
the fetus than in the fully formed child, he reasoned that it provides
the nutrition that permits the rest of the body to grow. In his formulation, the placenta supplies the maternal blood to the embryonic liver,
which purifies it, so that it can then go out via the great veins to nourish the developing body and support its growth. The rest of the body,
he believed, is formed from the liver, which is therefore its organ of
growth and nutrition. According to his thesis, the wastes left after purification are discharged into the fetal gallbladder.

With Galenic physiology assigning such an important role to the liver, it is no wonder that the maintenance of the organ's health preoccupied physicians throughout the Middle Ages and into the Renaissance. A large body of literature exists attesting to the many hepatic fluctuations that were thought by doctors of those times to produce illness. All of the abnormalities were in one way or another attributed to various imbalances in the humors. Although a wide variety of the ancient Hippocratic therapies were employed to treat these diseases—such as diet, baths, purging, puking, massage, changes of place or type of living, bloodletting, and even occasionally some form of surgery—the mainstay was drug therapy. Study of medieval texts reveals the names and constituents of large numbers of medications for presumed hepatic malfunctions, the vast majority of which were of plant origin.

In all, some two hundred individual plant species were said to have beneficial effects on the liver, sometimes given alone and sometimes as one of a prescription of many ingredients. A vast majority of the constituents of these complicated prescriptions were botanical, but a few might be animal or mineral. In recognition of their basis in the second-century physician's theories, the term *galenical* came to be used in reference to a prescription, whether for liver disease or anything else, of many plant substances. The use of galenicals, under that name, persisted until as late as the early twentieth century. They are no longer called by that old-fashioned designation, but some of the remedies of present-day nature healers and others are essentially the same thing, or at least very similar. Although evidence of their usefulness is often no less tenuous than is that of the medieval recipes, certain of their ingredients have from time to time proven to be effective, and sometimes even for the very purposes for which they were traditionally employed.

A brief listing of some of the herbal remedies used against presumed liver ailments indicates that some remain essential ingredients even today (although not necessarily for hepatic indispositions and not necessarily effective) in the therapies used in folk and traditional medicine, as well as those of today's natural healers. Among them are:

fennel, rue, asparagus, oregano, St. John's wort, black nightshade, barberry, camphor, citron, rose, sandalwood, laurel, endive, camomile, and absinthe. Of these, the one most heralded nowadays is St. John's wort, whose efficacy in cases of mild depression (thought for almost two millennia to be due to an excess of black bile, or *melas chole,* whence "melancholy") has not only withstood the test of time but is now sufficiently documented that it is frequently prescribed by psychiatrists.

Although a few of the liver diseases for which these herbs were believed to be efficacious might be recognized by a modern physician, the meaning of the old terminology is in almost all ways quite different from how the same words are used today. For example, the most commonly diagnosed hepatic problems were thought to be caused by an obstruction or blockage of the liver or its passages. We have no way of knowing what this actually meant, but we can be sure that it does not refer to the same entity now known as obstructive jaundice, in which a stone or tumor blocks the bile ducts. Various plant species, all now recognized to increase the flow of urine, were ingredients of prescriptions recommended to clear the "obstruction."

Other commonly diagnosed hepatic diseases of yore fall into several categories: the liver is thought to require purification; the liver is hot; the liver is hard; the liver is weak; the liver is dry; the liver contains a tumor. (It should not be thought that this latter diagnosis actually meant that a tumor was present, merely that the physician, for whatever reason, *thought* it was. Rarely could it be proven.)

Reliance on herbal remedies may be seen as a manifestation of the concept that man is at one with the natural forces around him; this follows not only from the near-universal beliefs of early civilizations concerning the importance of harmony between the microcosm and macrocosm but is also the product of the ancient Hippocratic emphasis on the healing power of nature—animal and plant merge into each other's domains. This kind of thinking pervaded medical diagnosis and therapy during all of the centuries that galenicals were a mainstay of treatment. The seventeenth-century metaphysical poet and divine George Herbert expressed in a few lines the accepted relationship between man, nature, and the cosmos, when he wrote:

Herbs gladly cure our flesh, because they
Find their acquaintance there.

More servants wait on man
Than he'll take notice of. In every path
He treads down that which doth befriend him
When sickness makes him pale and wan.
O mighty love! Man is one world, and hath

Another to attend him.

Herbert chose the word *acquaintance* advisedly, since the presumed efficacy of many of the herbal remedies was thought to be due to the symbolic relationship between the appearance of the botanical and the disease or the organ in which it manifested itself. Several of the plants that were commonly employed in cases of liver disease, for example, have yellow blossoms; absinthe, used in the treatment of jaundice, is one of them. This practice became codified in a principle known as the doctrine of signatures, by which it was taught that herbal remedies might be prescribed because they resemble the organ being treated or were in some way a reflection of the disease. Based on this formulation, for example, certain trilobed plants were used against liver disease during the long period when it was thought that the human liver had three lobes. The magical component has not to this day been completely expunged from the pharmacopeia of the herbalists, even if many of them are unaware of the basis of its traditional usage.

It was in resistance to this background of inherited hocus-pocus that the reform of medical theory began to show some early advances in the sixteenth and seventeenth centuries. By far the most prominent of the early reformers was an eccentric genius born in 1493 and known to the ages as Paracelsus, a name he gave himself.

Paracelsus was the most original medical thinker since Galen. His career so epitomizes the characteristic ways in which magic, religion, and medical science have intertwined themselves that he has forced his way into the narrative at this juncture. In typically confrontational Paracelsian fashion, he does not care a whit that this discussion is about the liver—he demands to be heard, and right now. It would be a mistake not to take advantage of his presence here. Though a temporary digression from our present immersion in matters hepatic, the story of his life cannot be left untold in a book that treats of the mythologies in the art of healing. He is the subject writ large, as we are about to see.

Though Paracelsus adhered to the belief that mystical God-motivated powers control biological processes in some grand scheme of microcosm and macrocosm, he nonetheless recognized that chemical principles underlie nature's functioning. Discarding the theory of humors, he thought of disease as less a generalized problem than a disorder of a specific organ. In this, he was disagreeing with one of the most basic principles of all previous medicine, enshrined since the time of Hippocrates but accepted long before. Physicians of that early era may have noted that symptoms manifest themselves in a single organ, but they were nevertheless convinced that this was merely the localized expression of a generalized process involving the entire body.

Paracelsus introduced a scheme of therapy based on chemicals rather than botanicals. But, having abandoned one principle of Galenic medicine, he reinvoked another, which had been honored only in the breach since the authoritarianism of Galen had set medical theory into a fixity of straitened traces: Experience and personal observation, he argued loudly, are the keys to understanding the body, not dogma and not the unthinking acceptance of what was found in books and handed down by tradition from one generation to the next.

Paracelsus's dual emphasis on observation and chemistry profoundly influenced some of the leading physicians of the generations following him, among whom was the aforementioned Jean Baptiste van Helmont. Van Helmont, while remaining as convinced as was Paracelsus of the hegemony of spiritual forces, would take chemical analysis to the next level and become the founder of the school that came to be called iatrochemistry. Iatrochemistry grew out of the doctrines of Paracelsus, which in turn owed a great deal to alchemy.

Alchemy was as much a philosophy as it was a product of the laboratory. Its underlying theory was the ancient principle that all matter is a unity, whether in the heavens or on earth, and each of the various forms of matter is endowed with its own spiritual being. It was yet another manifestation of the notion that the microcosm of a human being is both a part of and a reflection of the macrocosm of the natural world and the heavens.

There being a single pure essence for all things, the goal of alchemy was to achieve the perfection that lies within metal or man. For metal, said the alchemists, this was gold; for man, it was a form of completeness represented by long life, redemption, and immortality.

Such concepts can be found in Indian Vedic texts as early as the tenth century B.C.E., and in Taoist thinking in the second century B.C.E. They were known also during the western classical period. From there, they can be traced to the beginnings of Arab alchemy in the eighth century C.E., and then to Western Europe.

Alchemy was hardly science. Although its practitioners designed and used complex laboratory apparatus, their theories were a mixture of magic, astrology, and the earliest forms of chemistry, made all the more confusing by deliberate attempts to keep their practices secret. But out of the mumbo jumbo of esoterica, concealment, and mysticism, some genuine chemical contributions came forth, including, for example, the discovery of alcohol and certain acids.

Amidst all the recondite supernaturalism of the sixteenth-century alchemists, there appeared—perhaps "exploded onto the scene" is a better description—Paracelsus, a man seemingly larger than life, who would become the transitional figure between the sorcery of their quasi science and the development of a real medical chemistry. The very name by which he was known proclaims his distinctiveness and provides tantalizing clues to the background against which he dared to challenge not only the fuzziness of alchemical theory but the theory of the two-thousand-year-old orthodox medicine as well.

Philippus Aureolus Theophrastus Bombastus von Hohenheim was the son of a Swiss-born physician and humanistic scholar who added Theophrastus to his only child's Christian name of Philippus to honor the memory of one of Aristotle's pupils. *Aureolus* means "golden haired," and seems to have been a nickname bestowed on the boy because of his appearance while young, but one wonders whether more was not implied about the fair-haired lad. As for *Bombastus*—we can only guess, although his personality in later life would certainly justify such an addition. As if this list of multisyllabic appellations was not sufficiently lengthy, our man, following the custom of many other Renaissance humanists, gave himself a Latin name, Paracelsus. Although he left no clue to his reasons for this choice, it has been theorized that he did it out of sheer—yes—bombast. Celsus had been a first-century Roman scholar who produced a three-book work that became the general reader's definitive encyclopedia of all then known about medicine; some say that Philippus Theophrastus chose his *nom de science,* as it were, as a statement that he had exceeded even the great Celsus.

When Paracelsus, as he has become universally known to the ages, was a schoolboy, his father practiced in the town of Villach in southern Austria, the site of several mines and a smelting works, as well as a school where young men were trained to oversee mining operations of gold, tin, mercury, and iron. Paracelsus had already developed the attitude toward education that he would carry throughout his life: Traditional patterns of schooling only serve to enforce traditional ideas; the world must be seen with a fresh view and eyes undimmed by reading the old texts; the secret of learning is the realization that founts of knowledge are everywhere around us, whether they be found in the words of beggars, miners, tradesmen, doctors, or little old ladies.

Paracelsus absorbed a great deal of what was then known of chemistry and metallurgy from his contacts at the school, and then continued to apply his educational theories even after he had obtained his degrees in liberal arts and medicine, probably at the universities of Vienna and Ferrara, in 1510 and 1516, respectively. This is to say that he traveled widely throughout Europe, supporting himself by practicing medicine and learning all he could from whomever he met. There is evidence that he lived in France, Spain, Portugal, the British Isles, Denmark, Sweden, Lithuania, and Poland, in addition to making shorter visits to Hungary, Romania, Croatia, Constantinople, Crete, and Alexandria, always refining his theories and validating them to his satisfaction at the bedside. Nor should it be thought that he had spent his university years only at Vienna and Ferrara. He went from one school to another during that time, seeking teachers—usually in vain—who would not disappoint him. At various times, he studied at the universities of Basel, Tübingen, Wittenberg, Leipzig, Heidelberg, and Cologne. Perhaps he should have added Peripateticus to his long list of names.

With his determination to escape the stifling hold of the Galen-inspired medical theories of his time, Paracelsus opened himself to the absorption of all that could be learned around him. It was not enough that he be a good physician—he must be so unencumbered by the straitjacketing theoretics of his peers that he could contemplate anew the basic mechanisms of disease. Not only had medical theory stagnated since Galen's time, but therapies were fixed into a rote pattern that allowed little flexibility for the individual physician to perceive the problems of the individual patient.

Despite his iconoclasm, Paracelsus accepted without question one of the major philosophical assumptions of his time: the microcosm/macrocosm thesis—man can only be understood by studying nature and God. He believed also in the distinctiveness of each person and the influence on disease of a patient's unique emotional and spiritual nature. Though ancient in origin, this latter idea was nevertheless inconsistent with the rigid scholasticisms with which the medicine of the time had become imbued. Also inconsistent with them was his certainty that there was still much to learn about human biology. This was a period in which physicians and scholars had convinced themselves that they had developed a complete system to explain health and disease, with only bits and pieces of the overall pattern yet to be filled in. Paracelsus vigorously denied that.

Well equipped to extract value from the alchemists' lore that even they did not know could be found in it, Paracelsus used the information he gleaned from their experiments to bring forth a goodly number of effective means of clinical treatment, including mercury for the still relatively new scourge of syphilis, a therapy he introduced in a publication in 1530 that was the best clinical description of the disease written up to that time. Though he raged at the generally worthless hodge-podge of herbal concoctions of his day, his attempts at therapeutic minimalizing were not always well conceived. Among his errors was the belief that small quantities of the substance thought to cause a disease were capable of curing it, a concept which centuries later would become one of the founding principles of homeopathy. But most importantly and fundamentally, he demonstrated that a comprehension of chemistry is the pathway toward understanding the body and treating disease.

Paracelsus became well known for some of his cures, among which, incidentally, are included those for mental diseases, which he treated by individualizing the medicines he prescribed, an idea virtually unheard of at the time. He became equally well known for his knowledge of surgery and his judgment about its indications. After saving the prominent Swiss printer Johannes Frobenius from a recommended amputation of his right foot, he followed up his triumph with the successful treatment of his patient's illustrious house guest, Erasmus. As a result of these two heralded coups, Paracelsus was called to be professor at the University of Basel in June of 1527 and to serve as municipal physician to the city.

At last, he would have a worthy forum in which to promote his ideas. But it was not to be. Paracelsus, ever the rebel, could not resist a demonstration of revolt, which his new colleagues quite naturally saw as a revolting demonstration. On arrival, the new professor almost immediately did two things that infuriated the entire faculty. The first was to announce his program for the new medicine, which he had printed and sent to the students, his new colleagues, and physicians elsewhere. Not even attempting to conceal his contempt for contemporary medical theory, he pointed out that the art of medicine had decayed:

> But we shall free it from its worst errors. Not by following that which those of old taught, but by our own observation of nature, confirmed by extensive practice and long experience. Who does not

know that most doctors today make terrible mistakes, greatly to the harm of their patients? Who does not know that this is because they cling too anxiously to the teachings of Hippocrates, Galen, Avicenna and others? . . . Day after day I will publicly elucidate for two hours, with great industry and to the great advantage of my hearers, books on practical and theoretical medicine, internal medicine, and surgery, books written by myself. I did not, like other medical writers, compile these books out of extracts from Hippocrates or Galen, but in ceaseless toil I created them anew, upon the foundation of experience, the supreme teacher of all things. If I want to prove anything, I shall not try to do it by quoting authorities, but by experiment and by reasoning thereon. If therefore, my dear readers, one of you should feel the impulse to penetrate these divine mysteries, if within a brief space of time he should want to fathom the depths of medicine, let him come to me at Basel, and he will find much more than I can utter in a few words. To express myself more plainly, let me say, by way of example, that I do not believe in the ancient doctrine of the complexions and the humours, which have been falsely supposed to account for all diseases. It is because these doctrines prevail that so few physicians have a precise knowledge of illnesses, their causes, and their critical days. I forbid you, therefore, to pass a facile judgment upon Theophrastus until you have heard him for yourselves. Farewell, and come with a good will to study our attempt to reform medicine.

As if this were not enough to alienate his fellow faculty members, Paracelsus found it necessary symbolically to cast out the men whose philosophies had so transfixed medieval and Renaissance medicine into the rigid patterns he decried. Three weeks after his appointment began, he publicly burned the books of Galen and the greatest of the Greek physician's Arabic successors, Avicenna, in front of the university. Martin Luther having less than seven years earlier consigned to the pyre a papal bull threatening his own excommunication, the comparison must not have escaped the onlookers.

If Paracelsus thought his dramatic act would herald the beginning of a new era of medical teaching, he was wrong. The faculty rose up against him to a man. Before long the students—who he was confidently assuming would side with him—had also become alienated, in part by their difficulty in understanding his ideas and in part also because supporting him would have meant abandoning their other faculty, a decision too dangerous to contemplate. And in addition, there was the problem of Paracelsus's personal habits. In his long years of traveling, he had become a heavy drinker accustomed to peppering his everyday speech with profanity and demeaning attacks on his fellow professors, delivered with a grandiosity that went even beyond the usual self-glorifying manner of the time. Not only was he slovenly in his dress, but he refused to wear the academic regalia that was the daily uniform of the faculty. He lasted precisely eight months in Basel. So outraged had his colleagues and students become by his infuriating behavior that he had to flee in the middle of the night because his life was in danger.

Once again, he returned to his travels. As before, he took his chemical apparatus everywhere he went, to do research and to prepare remedies for his patients. His career was far from over and much work remained to be done, including the contribution to the treatment of syphilis noted above. His grandiosity was not lessened by his Basel experience; he continued to consider himself the only man who had ever truly understood disease and its treatment. Some three years after his academic debacle, he wrote in the preface to one of his essays:

> Avicenna, Galen, Rhazes, Montagnana, Mesue, and others: after me, and I not after you! Ye of Paris, ye of Montpellier, ye of Swabia, ye of Meissen, ye of Cologne, ye of Vienna, and those who dwell on the Danube and the Rhine, ye islands on the sea, thou Italy, thou Dalmatia, thou Sarmatia, thou Athens, ye Greeks, ye Arabs, ye Israelites: after me, and not I after you! Even in the remotest corner there will be none of you on whom the dogs will not pis. But I shall be monarch and mine will be the monarchy, and I shall lead the monarchy; gird your loins.

Raging, misunderstood, and scorned as he was—withal, Paracelsus perceived a truth that would one day become the foundation stone of medicine: Biological processes are nothing other than the result of physicochemical reactions. As he put it, "Nature is the arch-chemist and we must imitate her, otherwise we are no more than kitchen-sluts." Though he wrote of spiritual factors in the substances he worked with, and of nonmaterial forces in their reactions, he was nevertheless the first person to point out the biochemical nature of nature.

The great medical innovator might have been forgotten after he died in 1541 (some say he was knifed to death in a tavern brawl, others that he succumbed to cancer), alone and impoverished at the age of forty-eight, but for the books he wrote and his influence on his too-few disciples, most particularly van Helmont. The father of iatro-chemistry and those who followed him took the investigational path that would, in time, lead to the abandonment of the notion of humors and the other impedimenta of Galenic medicine. By pursuing a form of research and of healing based on chemical principles, they would promulgate a system that would eventually lead to the great accomplishments of modern medicine.

The ancient theoretical formulations would gradually be abandoned, the old books would become curiosities, and—though it took the better part of three centuries to accomplish it—the reliance on mysticism would eventually fade. Though a believer in the occult and a mystic himself—and certainly a vitalist (it should not be forgotten that the concept of *archei* was his invention)—Paracelsus sowed the seeds of biochemistry, physiology, and ultimately molecular medicine. But so paradoxical is his legacy that some remember him as an initiator of the changes that would lead to a scientific approach to disease, while others hail him as a hero of alternative medicine, mystical healing systems, and even homeopathy.

There does seem to be truth in both viewpoints. There can be no doubt that Paracelsus introduced the concept of chemistry into medicine, but his basic assumption was that it is not the element or compound itself—his big three were mercury, sulfur, and salt—but certain undefinable and experimentally unverifiable (to his mind, spiritual) qualities within it that determine its effect on the body. Moreover, like so many physicians of his time he was a believer in the so-called doctrine of signatures referred to earlier, in which the appearance of certain natural substances foretold their qualities in human physiology. For example, the word *orchid* derives from the Greek *orchis,* meaning "like a testicle," because the plant's ball-shaped double root resembles two testicles. To Paracelsus, this meant that the plant was capable of curing venereal diseases.

This kind of magical thinking is characteristic of the confusion that was rampant in those transitional centuries. Although viewing medical practice on the one hand as an attempt to understand and influence natural processes, Paracelsus was on the other convinced that those same natural processes were comprehensible through symbolic factors, based on his belief that the underlying essence of all life force is spiritual in nature. No matter the vigorous attempts by modern advocates of certain alternative healing practices to provide verifiable explanations for their various formulas—compelled as they are by the scientific age in which we live—such explanations are, like those of Paracelsus, too often without any possibility of experimental justification; those predisposed to accept them must do so with the full acknowledgment that these practices are based on a belief system that has thus far only incompletely withstood the objective eye of scientific validation. This does not mean, of course, that researchers should cease their explorations of the validity of certain claims, but adherents of folk and traditional forms of healing must acknowledge that their convictions are based on millennia-old beliefs that in many cases are not susceptible to proof.

And so Paracelsus must be seen not only as a transitional figure but also as a contradictory one. He advocated the study of nature while endowing nature with some of the same supernatural qualities as do shamans and witch doctors; he championed experience over theory as the great teacher, but allowed his spiritualistic formulations to determine the interpretation of his experience; he disavowed the dogmatic writings of the Galenists, while demanding rigid acceptance of his own dogmas; he disparaged those who obtained their learning from books, and yet insisted that the books he wrote contained the only truths. All in all, Paracelsus attacked authority, maintaining that only *his* authority was valid.

In one major characteristic, Paracelsus seems most like his predecessors; in another, he pointed the way toward a new medicine. His similarity with those who came before lies in his certainty that he had discovered an overarching system of medicine. Small details were to be filled in with more experiments and more experience, but he was certain that he had achieved an essential understanding of the processes of health and disease. In this, he was like the advocates of traditional medicine who today regard him as their hero. One of the several characteristics that differentiate science from all other ways of understanding nature is that the former is reductionist in the sense that small observations are the key to understanding; each of them must be interpreted under its own conditions and taken on its own terms. Every seeming certainty is subject to reevaluation and change. Except in their general approach of observation, hypothesis, experimental verification, and theory, scientists believe in no eternal verities. Everything is subject to alteration when new information becomes available. The greenest graduate student may demolish a theory promulgated by the holder of an endowed chair—or even a Nobelist. Other than the discoverable laws of physics and chemistry, no fixed overarching system exists into which all observed phenomena fit, and by which they can be explained.

Traditional systems, on the other hand, *begin* with an inherited explanation into which all observable patterns must be accommodated. They are accepted by their adherents as being eternally all-inclusive and all-explanatory. They are not constantly subjected to the scrutiny, skeptical reevaluation, and even iconoclastic thinking that characterize the scientific mind; great portions, if not frankly all, of their principles are accepted without the rigorous demand for evidence required by science. They are take-it-or-leave-it, all-or-nothing phenomena. Most important: traditional medicine is so called because it is based on tradition; the only evidence universally required by its exponents is that it has always been done this way; it has been handed down to generation after generation and it is accepted. Scientific medicine is ever new, ever changing, ever being challenged. The hoary hand of tradition has no grip on it—at least ideally.

It was in Paracelsus's conviction that he was introducing an all-explaining medicine that he was most like those who preceded him. It was in his insistence, regardless of its mystical bias, that chemistry lay at the basis of biology that he was a harbinger of a new kind of healing. To study the details of chemical reactions required a certain objectivity of viewpoint. Though followers like van Helmont were unable to free themselves of spiritual explanations for some of the phenomena they witnessed in the laboratory, they did learn the value of carefully recorded observations, measurements, and experiments. This kind of thinking would lead to new and real contributions.

A case in point was the first reliable textbook of anatomy based on actual dissections, published in a beautifully illustrated volume by a twenty-eight-year-old Belgian, Andreas Vesalius, in 1543. Another was William Harvey's discovery of the circulation of the blood less than a century later. Both based their publications on meticulous records of laboratory studies, done without regard to the fixed opinions of their predecessors. In Harvey's case, this required repeated experiments, careful measurements, and interpretations based on mechanics. In Vesalius's, it meant protracted periods of dangerous and gruesome work on decaying corpses to make exacting observations that repeatedly differed from the canonized writ that appeared in every text of his time. The few speculations these two men allowed themselves arose from their notions of probability. Even by today's standards, their contributions were remarkable. By the standards of their time, they were astonishing.

In the hands of Vesalius and Harvey, it was the body itself that was to be researched. After them, the purpose of medical studies was directed at what Vesalius referred to when he entitled his monumental book *De humani corporis fabrica* ("On the Workings of the Human Body"). In reference to the liver, the first effect of his contribution was a volume that appeared in 1654, called *Anatomia hepatis*, by Francis

Glisson, Regius Professor of Physic [Medicine] at Cambridge. By boiling the organ until its substance was soft enough to be wiped away, the author was able to identify some of its many ductal structures and a fine fibrous envelope by which the liver is encased, known since that time as Glisson's capsule. As seemingly tenuous as it is, this very thin layer nevertheless has sufficient strength that it was able to hold the stitches I used to close the cut edges of Harriet Dale's liver.

As Glisson repeatedly studied the livers of animals, he came to the conclusion that the flow of bile is not uniform, but rather that it intermittently increases, apparently in response to some stimulus. Following from these observations, he conceived of the idea that irritation of the gallbladder and bile ducts was the stimulus in question, leading him to a theory that was to remain popular for centuries. It was Glisson's notion that irritability is an inherent property of all living tissue and was the cause of the movements of muscle. Not only that, but it was also the cause of life itself; without irritability, life cannot exist.

So far, so good. In fact, Glisson's theory is consistent in certain ways with present-day physiological thought, even if backwards: today, irritability—we speak actually of responsiveness—is recognized to be a function of living tissue; the tissue is responsive because it is alive. To Glisson, it was the metaphysical property of irritability that gave life to tissue. So even this distinguished physician—he was a president of the Royal College of Physicians and one of the founders of the Royal Society—could not keep himself from interjecting a bit of supernaturalism or vitalism into his theory. Irritability became, in his mind, related to the soul, and therefore a property invested with nonmaterial qualities. Thus did yet another otherwise objective scientist fall in line with those seduced by the supernal. He was a man of his time, who could not shed the preconceptions of his era.

Not until the era that historians call the modern period were researchers able to separate themselves entirely from vitalistic theory. One of the contributing factors to the turn from supernaturalism was a gradual rejection of the notion that the promulgation of great theories was the road to understanding. When medical science became less ambitious, it also became more productive. One of the earliest exponents of "thinking smaller" was François Magendie of Bordeaux (1783–1855), who has been called the pioneer of experimental physiology. His was an attitude of minuteness and exactness of observation rather than expansiveness of doctrine. Despairing of the usefulness of generalizations, he sought to make isolated observations with particularity, rather than creating a systematic theory of everything. He was fond of referring to himself, in fact, as a *chiffonier,* a ragpicker, taking up whatever he could as he wandered through the scientific terrain. He collected observations and experiments in anticipation of a usefulness they might later prove to have.

Magendie exerted a profound influence on the young Claude Bernard, then a junior physician studying with him at the Collège de France in Paris. So impressed was Bernard with his mentor's approach to gathering biological information that he saw the pre-Magendie centuries as one long period of what he called *rêverie systématique,* or "systematic dreaming," rather than real science.

Of the tendency toward prejudged and sometimes far-fetched interpretations of experimental findings that characterized too much of scientific thinking (and to an extent still does), Bernard would later write:

> Put off your imagination, as you take off your overcoat, when you enter the laboratory; but put it on again, as you do your overcoat, when you leave the laboratory. Before the experiment and between whiles, let your imagination wrap you round; put it right away from you during the experiment lest it hinder your powers of observation.

Of course, he was pointing out, imagination is important to a researcher, else he could not conceive of the new hypotheses that must be tested by the imaginative use of experiment. But while that experiment is being done, only the detached observer can see the events that are truly unfolding before his eyes. Scientific imagination, he said, must be based on scientifically derived evidence.

When Bernard turned his considerable talents to studying the liver, he came up with the discovery, in the late 1850s, that one of the major functions of that organ is to store carbohydrate so that it is readily available when the body needs an energy source; in a sense, the liver is like a storage battery. It was later found that a hormone, insulin, stimulates the liver to take glucose from the bloodstream and convert it into the complex sugar molecule called glycogen. When required, the liver converts its stored glycogen back into glucose to provide energy for immediate use. Not only that, but the organ manufactures additional glucose from the building blocks of protein, called amino acids.

The liver may not have proven to be the seat of life, but it was rapidly revealing itself to have a far more complex range of jobs than anyone had foreseen. Following on the work of Bernard, others discovered many new things about the organ, with no necessity of invoking magic to explain them. In time, its methods of making bile were elucidated, as were certain contributions it makes to immunity, including its ability to detoxify, filter, and sanitize various substances in the bloodstream. We now know how it makes the proteins that circulate in the blood plasma, manufactures cholesterol and regulates its level in the blood, and in general provides ways for fats, proteins, and carbohydrates to become converted one into another. In a pinch, it can even make blood cells, but *only* in a pinch. Galen would not have been pleased to know that the corpuscles giving the blood its very color are formed in the hollow centers of bones, with the liver taking part only when there is massive hemorrhage or destruction of the marrow, events unlikely to happen in the life of any given individual. Not only Galen, in fact, but every physician of an earlier time who used metaphysics and pure invention to fill the gaps in his knowledge would be astonished at what has been discovered by science. With regard to the liver, they would be flabbergasted.

The tradition of calling on supernature as the basis for phenomena still unexplained by science is an old habit of mankind, but in the long run a counterproductive one. It does us no honor. Remaining gaps in current knowledge are not evidence for the existence of God. The god of the gaps is not a god worth worshiping. Science and religion are not at odds—they explain two separate realms of human experience. The faithful need no justification for their faith. It is enough that they believe. And God should not be invoked in place of knowledge not yet discovered.

CHAPTER SIX

THE SPLEEN: ORGAN OF MYSTERY, ORGAN OF MELANCHOLY

EVERY career, every job, has its unstated perks. The actor gets free theater tickets; the carpenter repairs his garage using nails and wood bought at a wholesaler's discount; the lawyer fires off letters without expense, perhaps threatening suit for any personal annoyance; the flight attendant travels all over the world at minimal expense. Who knows how many public officials have had their parking tickets fixed?

Even semiskilled garment workers have their own special deals. My father spent most of his adult years hunched over a sewing machine in the poorly lit warrens of a succession of small dress manufacturers on Seventh Avenue in Manhattan, barely earning a living at the minimal piece-goods wages he was grudgingly paid by demanding bosses. But every few years, on those rare occasions when one of his sons absolutely had to have a new pair of pants or even a suit to replace one outgrown or threadbare, Pop always seemed to know someone who knew someone—and maybe that someone knew someone else. A sequence of contacts was made, and my brother Harvey and I would be taken—invariably on a Saturday morning—to one of those buzzingly busy lofts where men's clothing (my father called it cludding) was created from large bolts of fabric lying all over the cluttered cutting tables.

Prices were always lower than wholesale in those manufacturing lofts, and the owners—being hard up for cash themselves—were predictably responsive to a bit of good-natured haggling, which was dignified by being called bargaining. The deals were made in the homely rhythms of colloquial Yiddish, and were consummated with a handshake and the exchange of cash. Choices among the garments were few, but the cludding never fit less than perfectly, because the final adjustments were completed on the spot and on the boy.

But no one enjoys more job-related perks than do doctors. We treat people who come to us from a vast panorama of occupations, and the opportunities for special privileges are endless; they go well beyond the specialness of the medical care that colleagues provide to our families. Patients like to express gratitude to their physicians with gifts that take a wide variety of forms, ranging from homemade cookies or a dozen freshly picked tomatoes to discounted prices on cars and the occasional "Hey, Doc, I can let you in on a great real estate deal in Bermuda." The mouths of some gift horses must be carefully inspected; I would guess that few physicians take advantage of offers like that last one. But even fewer are likely to turn their backs on the chance to fly their families to Europe without cost, and I among the least likely of all. Thanks to a spleen, I once had it within my grasp. Or so it seemed.

These days, the medical needs of the students, faculty, and employees of Yale University are seen to by a large corporate entity called the Yale Health Plan. This sprawling enterprise was preceded by a much simpler system in which all salaried personnel chose health insurance and their own doctors, while the students were cared for by a small cadre of physicians employed by the university. When specialty services, such as surgery, were required, they were contracted to one of a group of clinical faculty of the medical school. In the early years of my practice, I was a member of that group.

Late one weekday afternoon during a fall semester in the mid-1960s, I stopped by the Yale Infirmary to check on an undergraduate who was recovering from an appendectomy. As I sat writing a note in his chart, one of the nurses asked me to look in on a sophomore who had dislocated his left shoulder a few hours earlier during an intramural soccer game. The problem, she said, was the severity of the boy's pain. The moonlighting medical resident on duty had ordered a standard oral painkiller, but "it's not even touching him, and I can't figure out why."

The infirmary occupied a large and rather grand three-story brick house built near the close of the nineteenth century by a prosperous New Haven family. Entering the spacious corner room being shared by the student with another undergraduate, I found him sitting upright in bed clutching his left shoulder with his right hand. Grimacing with pain, he told me that he had crashed into another player as the two were running in opposite directions at top speed. On being asked to demonstrate the point of collision, he lowered his hand from the painful shoulder and placed its flattened palm on the rib margin between his lower chest and upper abdomen. "I must have hit my shoulder when I fell," he said, by way of explaining the discrepancy between the pain and its putative cause.

"Must have? But aren't you sure?"

"I just assumed that's what happened. How else could I have dislocated it?"

When I examined the shoulder, it was perfectly normal. Not only did it appear unscathed by the fall but it was not tender to firm pressure. The boy could move his arm in any direction I asked him to.

"What makes you so sure it's dislocated?"

"I'm positive, because of the pain. You know, I've had this problem once before, and it was a lot like what I'm feeling now."

"A lot?"

"Well, it was a long time ago."

The student, whom I'll call Jim Bornemann, had been brought to the infirmary by a teammate at about 5:00 P.M., a few minutes after the attending physician on duty left for the day. The moonlighting Yale–New Haven Hospital resident, arriving about ten minutes later, had been busily making rounds, beginning on the third floor and wending his gradual way from room to room. He had not yet seen Jim, who had arrived at the infirmary, told the nurses he had a dislocated shoulder, and been put right to bed as soon as his admission blood count was drawn and a urine specimen taken. On being told about the new admission, the young doctor ordered pain medication, which was administered before the nurses rejoined the team on rounds. In the shuffle, no one had yet had the opportunity to examine Jim.

I asked the boy if he hurt anywhere else.

"Sure—right where I was hit." He ran his left hand lightly across his upper abdomen, a move he certainly could not have made so thoughtlessly had he actually suffered a shoulder dislocation. When I asked him to touch one finger to the most painful spot in the shoulder, he moved his hand unerringly to its very top, near the lateral end of the collarbone. The correct diagnosis became clear when I asked him to tell me when the discomfort had begun.

"Oh, about fifteen minutes after I was hit. Not right away, for some reason."

"The reason is probably that you've ruptured your spleen. Let's have you lie down and I'll examine your belly."

"I can't lie down. It makes the pain a lot worse."

"Well, that clinches it."

I listened to his abdomen with my stethoscope and heard not a sound. When I had convinced him to lie flat enough, I felt his abdominal wall. It was hard, and a little tender when I pressed into the left side. All of this meant that something was irritating the inside of the abdominal cavity. Without a doubt, it was blood.

I explained to Jim the principle of referred pain, in which discomfort is felt in an area even though its actual cause is somewhere else. In early embryological development, the diaphragm originates in the lower part of the neck and only later migrates downward. Accordingly, its sensory nerves arise from the same part of the spinal cord as do the nerves carrying sensation from the top of the shoulder. Pain that is actually caused by irritation of the diaphragm is felt as pain in the shoulder. This explains why Jim thought he had a dislocation. Because the upright position allows the injured spleen to drop away from the diaphragm just a bit, it lessens the pain.

It was just at this point that the medical student on duty in the small basement lab phoned upstairs to report that Jim's white blood cell count was somewhat high, and he had a marked elevation in the neutrophils, the cells that increase in the presence of acute inflammation anywhere in the body. Also, the red cell count was a bit low. There could now be no question about the diagnosis. I called Jim's mother in a suburb of Chicago and told her the details of her son's situation. His slowly bleeding spleen would have to be removed within the next few hours, before the blood pressure began to drop and he went into shock. She agreed to the planned operation and told me that she and Jim's father would be arriving in New Haven as soon as they could get on a plane. As I would later discover, getting on a plane was no problem for the Bornemanns, since Jim's father was the vice president in charge of a major division of one of America's largest airlines. They arrived in town by midnight.

Jim dressed and I took him directly to the Yale–New Haven Hospital in my car. Though he must have been frightened, he adopted an air of stoic determination. The fascination of the bustling that took place around him when we arrived at the emergency room served as something of a distraction, and the anxiety may have been further lessened by the attentions of several attractive nursing students among the team hurriedly preparing him for the operating room. Within an hour of arrival at the hospital, my young patient had been anesthetized and I was ready to begin the operation.

On opening Jim's abdomen, I found that the rupture had occurred at the very top of the spleen, where a jagged crack in the organ's substance was plugged by a large mushy clot that was preventing further brisk hemorrhage. Although there was a bit of ooze still leaking through the base of the clot, the rapid phase of the bleeding had been stopped by the pressure of the coagulum filling the splenic laceration. There were about two pints of fresh blood in the abdominal cavity. I removed the spleen without undue difficulty and closed the abdomen. My patient awakened rapidly from the anesthesia and had a perfectly smooth postoperative course. He spent part of his recovery period in the same infirmary room where I had found him sitting bolt upright and clutching his shoulder.

Needless to say, Jim's parents were enormously pleased and deeply grateful. They were particularly impressed with the way the diagnosis was made and the expeditiousness with which the situation had been happily resolved. My attempts to explain to them that any reasonably competent surgeon would have done the same were heard as the protestations of a modest man, a charge which few who know me would ever think to make. Mrs. Bornemann stayed on until after her son was discharged from the hospital back to the infirmary, but her husband returned to Chicago a few days after the operation, certain that his son's life had been saved by a surgical miracle worker too reticent to accept credit. Nothing I said could convince him otherwise. Before he left, he took me aside and told me to be sure to contact him should I have any future plans for international travel. He pressed his business card into my hand, which proved not unwilling to accept it.

I assured Mr. Bornemann that I would be in touch with him. I had been planning a visit to London for the coming spring, with my wife and two young children. "Just call or write me," he said, with his last firm handclasp before rushing back to his busy office in Chicago. "I'll take care of everything—personally."

About two months before my planned visit, I did call my benefactor's office but never got past whoever picked up the phone, even after several attempts. Finally, I wrote a letter. The reply came promptly:

Dear Dr. Nuland,

Mr. Bornemann is pleased to hear that you are planning to use *** Airlines as your carrier to London. He has asked me to send you our company's enclosed travel brochures. On behalf of *** Airlines, he

sincerely wishes you and your family a pleasant journey. We hope we
can serve your travel needs again, at some time in the future.

With all good wishes,

Susan Pseudonym

Secretary to John W. Bornemann

A few colorful airline leaflets were in the envelope, of the sort avail-
able in every travel agency. I never heard anything further from Mr.
Bornemann. Three weeks later, I bought four full-price tickets to
London—on another airline.

THE story of Jim Bornemann describes only one of many colorful experiences I have had with the spleen, during a long career in which
the organ has figured prominently among my surgical interests. The
functions of the spleen; diseases of the spleen; surgery of the spleen;
the history of the spleen; the legends and lore of the spleen—each
of them has occupied my thoughts in many ways over the years.
Somewhere in the middle of my professional life, I discovered that the
spleen was involved with my very name.

The first action we are likely to take when a book of name deriva-
tions chances to fall into our hand is to look ourselves up. Most Janes
and Georges stop doing this after the first two or three searches, because they have by then ascertained the origin of their names and
nothing new is to be learned about them. But for those of us on whom
obscure and therefore rarely listed names have been inflicted, the
chase must often continue over a period of years, until a source is finally found that solves the mystery.

In the unlikely event that anyone named Sherwin is reading this
book, be advised that the very sound you hated as a child and have
come to rather like as an adult is derived from the Welsh for "shearing
the wind." This refers not to flatulence but to speed. To a Welshman,
a shearer of the wind—Sherwin—is a fast runner.

Kids being what they are, boys who carry a monicker like Sherwin
are unlikely to proceed far into adolescence without experiencing at

least an occasional taunt or tease. In the Bronx where I grew up, taunting and teasing led not infrequently to punching and wrestling, sometimes preceded by a chase in which the jeerer had to be caught by the jeeree before the pummeling could begin. This meant, of course, that a Sherwin not only had to live up to his name by being a fast runner but it was also incumbent on him that he be a good fighter. My problem, magnified by the generally confrontational Bronx of my childhood and adolescence, can be simply expressed: I was neither a fast runner nor a good fighter.

I would have given anything to be a speedy kid, even my spleen. Such a statement is not as far-fetched as it seems; the idea of giving up one's spleen in order to become a fast runner has a long and honorable history. At least since the days of ancient Greece, there have been those who believed that removal of the spleen, nowadays called splenectomy, is the key to fast running. Very likely, some athletes still believe this. Albeit obscure and rarely heard nowadays, an old French expression refers to it: *courir comme un dératé,* to run like a person despleened. My Cassell's French dictionary defines the phrase as "to run like a greyhound."

Like everything else about the early conceptions of splenic function, the origin of this particular bit of fantasy is shrouded in mystery, but there are a few clues. In the texts of the Hippocratic period there is frequent mention of the symptoms of a disease we now recognize as malaria, particularly prevalent in marshy locations such as were common in Greece and around Rome. Splenomegaly, or enlargement of the spleen, being a common finding in people with malaria, a number of ancient medical writings describe ways to shrink the offending organ, whose excessive size could cause problems ranging from mere discomfort to serious disability. In *De medicina,* his encyclopedic review of all then known about the art of healing, the Roman scholar Celsus attributed "pain and some difficulty in walking fast or running" to splenomegaly. Like many medical writers before him, Celsus provided a long list of remedies by which the organ might be shrunk, ranging from "anointings and rubbings" to imbibing any of a number of preparations made up of various vegetable or herbal ingredients. For a modern reader, one of his most curious suggestions is that the splenomegalic patient drink "water in which a blacksmith has from time to time dipped his red-hot irons; since the water especially reduces the spleen. For it has been observed that animals reared by our blacksmiths, have small spleens." Although Celsus provided no documentation for his assertion about the smiths' horses, many thousands of desperate patients must surely have taken his advice nevertheless.

Pliny the Elder, writing at about the same time, was another of those who commented on the spleen's role in slowing runners, telling his no-doubt gullible readers that athletes sometimes had the organ removed. Not only enlarged spleens were an indication for this, he wrote, but apparently any spleen at all: "This member hath a propertie by itself sometimes, to hinder a man's running: whereupon professed runners in the race that be troubled with the splene have a device to burne and waste it with a hot iron. . . . They say that the splene may be taken out of the body by way of incision, and yet the creature lives nevertheless."

It must be assumed that by "creature," Pliny meant an animal. Still, unverifiable reports do exist of attempts at splenectomy in young men. Although the likelihood is minuscule that even a healthy athlete could have survived such an operation, whether by hot iron or incision, references to it being done for this purpose are occasionally to be found in texts written hundreds of years before Pliny, as are comments about the role of even a healthy spleen being an impediment to speed.

The belief that splenectomy would allow people to run faster is enshrined in Talmudic literature as a comment on a passage from the biblical text of I Kings. Its appearance there is doubtless a reflection of the notion's widespread acceptance in the medical lore of the time, between the second and fourth centuries C.E. As King David lay dying, his son by Haggith, Adonijah, attempted to seize the throne before Solomon could ascend to it. "[H]e prepared him chariots and horsemen, and fifty men to run before him" (I Kings 1:5). In commenting on the biblical passage, the Babylonian Talmud states that the significant thing about these men is that all of them had had their spleens removed, which later rabbinic authorities interpreted as meaning that they were accordingly made swifter by the operation. Like other writings of the time that take up matters of health and nature, the Talmud also contains recipes for oral concoctions said to shrink the spleen.

Physicians as late as the seventeenth century—including as esteemed an authority as the illustrious William Harvey, whose discovery of the circulation of the blood is considered the greatest medical advance of all time—repeated unconfirmed reports that mail carriers in Turkey were having their spleens removed in order to facilitate running from place to place. Giving credence to such a possibility was a widely circulated description by the Neapolitan surgeon Leonardo Fioravanti of a successful operation that had been done in 1549, at which he assisted a colleague named Andriano Zaccarello in removing a massively enlarged spleen from a twenty-four-year-old Greek woman. Because Fioravanti's writings were very popular among physicians, the splenectomy story was widely circulated as evidence that the operation could be done. Most probably, however, what the two surgeons removed was not a spleen at all. Although Fioravanti described the excised specimen as being hard and cancerous in appearance, surgeons who read his report in later centuries believed that the operation was in fact the excision of a huge cyst of the ovary, a procedure much less demanding than splenectomy, on both patient and surgeon.

Very likely, the ancients reasoned that the problems caused by an enlarged spleen were only a magnification of the effects of having even a perfectly healthy spleen. To them, it must have made sense that the presence of a spleen, abnormal or not, slowed a man down. But there may have been an additional factor in the equation of spleen equals impediment to speed. The upper abdominal discomfort familiarly known as a stitch, noted by many people after the unaccustomed exertion of running some distance is—if my personal experience and anecdotal reports are to be believed—most commonly felt just below the front of the rib margin, usually on the left where the organ in question is located. Perhaps this should be added to the reasons why the spleen bore for at least two millennia its undeserved reputation as an inhibitor of velocity. Although there appears to be no absolutely verifiable documentation of human splenectomy until the early nineteenth century, it is impossible not to wonder how many young athletes died in ill-conceived attempts to remove the organ.

The fancy that despleening a man allows him to run faster is no more outlandish than are most of the beliefs that have characterized the history of an organ that was until relatively recent times an enigma to every authority who wrote about it. It was with good reason that Galen called the spleen *plenum mysterii organum,* "the organ full of mystery," and described its function with an amalgam of unsubstantiated theory inherited from his medical forebears, to which he added his own imaginings, presented—like all his writings—as though he were certain of their unalterable truth.

Among the most common twice-told tales of my medical school days is the apocryphal one said to have been set in the 1920s in which Dr. Milton Winternitz, the Yale dean and professor of pathology, one day called on an unprepared student to describe the functions of the spleen. Eager to cover the tracks of his ignorance in the forbidding presence of a teacher renowned for both toughness and sarcasm, the young man blurted out, "Oh—I know them all, yes I do, Dr. Winternitz. In fact, I was reading about the spleen just last night and I knew all there is to know about it, but I'm drawing a blank. I've forgotten everything!"

To which the sardonically sneering Winternitz is said to have replied, "Why, what a great loss to medical science. Just think—the only person in history ever to know what the spleen does, and he's forgotten it!" My guess is that every medical school has its own version of this story, even if the caustic wit of Winternitz was unique to New Haven. "What the spleen does" puzzled medical thinkers for more than two thousand years.

In the earliest of Hippocratic writings, the spleen was said to draw water from the body, thereby preventing any illness thought to be caused by water's excess. Plato, too, who was a contemporary of Hippocrates, saw the spleen as an organ of purification, cleansing the entire body of contaminants, but mainly those originating in the liver. In later Hippocratic texts, the water and the impure material are replaced by the humor called black bile, with the spleen thought to be both its source and its sink. When Galen came along some four hundred years later and codified medicine, he firmed up the earlier constructs by permanently assigning to the spleen the primary role in purging the body of any excess of the dark humor. According to him, the spleen is either the source or the first repository of black bile after its origin in the liver as a by-product of the manufacture of blood.

As with the other three humors, the sighting of black bile escaping the confines of the body was understood to be a sign of sickness. In fact, its visible presence was thought to be a finding more grave than even the overt appearance of blood, yellow bile, or phlegm, which were evident in hemorrhage, bilious vomiting, or a runny nose, respectively. One of the counsels in Hippocrates's *Aphorisms* declares, "If black bile be evacuated upwards or downwards, at the commencement of a disease, it is a fatal symptom."

The more one studies Greek and Roman writings about the spleen and black bile, the more inescapable becomes the conclusion that the ancients never quite knew what to make of either the organ or the humor associated with it. They could easily fit the stomach, liver, and intestines into their worldview of digestion and blood production, and the pancreas was so deeply buried in the back of the abdomen that it seemed not to need explaining, but the spleen—what could its function possibly be? Why is it positioned where it is, resting against the great lateral curve of the pillowy stomach and sheltered so securely within the gentle arc of the overlying ribs as though to keep it safe; as though it has some supreme importance to our lives; as though it must be protected against any possible harm? And what could that great importance be, if some authorities recommended its removal with the only consequence being an improvement in a man's ability to run? When things are not clear, the temptation to make up something out of whole cloth is irresistible, especially in a culture where every biological circumstance was believed to have come about for some specific reason.

Aristotle, who was a teenager when Hippocrates died, had his own ideas. He was much impressed with the fact that one side of an animal is more or less a mirror image of the other. He believed this bilaterality to be due to the necessity that the organs of locomotion be equalized. So, therefore, must all other structures. To him, "[T]he spleen looks rather like a bastard liver, . . . [T]he liver is patently double, and the larger part of it [the actual liver] tends to lie towards the right, the smaller [the spleen] towards the left." Further, "The spleen owes its existence to the liver being placed somewhat over to the right-hand side of the body. This makes the spleen a necessity in a way." In other words, the spleen does what the liver does, and is its equivalent on the opposite side of the body. Aristotle believed that it lies where it lies in order to be consistent with the principle of symmetry and bilaterality of the body, as exemplified in the upper and lower extremities.

Half a millennium later, Galen made his unchallengeable declaration that the spleen "is the instrument that eliminates the thick earthy humors formed in the liver. It attracts them [via the splenic and portal veins, shown by later anatomists to carry blood in precisely the opposite direction that Galen thought, namely from spleen to liver], and when it has done so, it does not immediately discharge them into the stomach, but first takes ample time to elaborate and alter them. . . . Those that have been altered into the juice most suitable for the viscus become nutriments to the spleen, but those that escape alteration there, that cannot be changed into the nature of thin, useful blood, and that are entirely unsuitable for nutriment are discharged by the spleen into another venous canal into the stomach." In other words, the residual black bile that cannot be used by the spleen or altered into blood passes from the spleen into the stomach. Galen recognized that the fluid in the stomach is acid, which he attributed to the presence of the black bile, which "tightens and draws together the stomach and compels it to clasp the food closely and retain it until it is completely concocted. This is the foresight with which Nature has arranged the discharge of the bilious residues."

Of course, none of this entire elaborate mechanism exists—Galen simply invented it. He was not only describing imaginary functions of the spleen but also telling his readers of the presence of a theoretical passageway that he insisted must carry the unused black bile directly into the stomach, where it causes a contraction that existed only in

Galen's mind. The medical world believed in this entire formulation for almost a millennium and a half, until much of it was demonstrated to be false by the Belgian anatomist Andreas Vesalius and others in the sixteenth century. Had anyone dared to question the anatomical formulations of the ancient voice of authority before then, the progress of medicine would certainly have taken quite a different course.

Galen's entire configuration of erroneous concepts makes sense only when seen as part of his overall scheme for fitting the spleen into his worldview of anatomy and physiology. To him, as to so many of his predecessors and successors, nature (he thought of it as Nature, virtually synonymous with the Divinity that had created the universe) made no structure in vain; he devoted his life to explaining the existence and purpose of every organ, its position and its function. On the occasions when he did this by carrying out valid, reproducible experiments and verifying his observations, he came to conclusions that can only be characterized as brilliant, especially considering the period in which they were made. But when no verifiable explanation of structure or function was forthcoming, he would invent one.

Galen probably tasted the contents of an animal's stomach and realized it was acid, in error attributing its acidity to the hypothetical black bile. Ironically, his erroneous interpretation of his presumed observation, whether made in this manner or not, would later find an echo in the work of Jean Baptiste van Helmont. In introducing his thesis that digestion in the stomach is not a process of coction as the ancients had said but rather is accomplished by acid, van Helmont had to explain how the acid got there in the first place. As radical an opponent of Galenic theory as he was, he nevertheless found it expedient to write that it is "borrowed from the spleen." The heritage of black bile lingered still.

It is fair to ask on what basis Galen or any of his predecessors were so sure that such a thing as black bile existed. Yellow bile, blood, and phlegm, after all, can be seen every time an animal is cut open—but black bile? What, precisely, is it and how did it first enter medical lore?

Very likely, the answer is to be found in the pervasive influence of Empedocles, the fifth-century B.C.E. Sicilian-born Greek philosopher whose wide intellectual heritage ranged from poetry to medicine. Because Empedocles was in his forties at the time Hippocrates is thought to have been born in 460 B.C.E., his authoritative teachings permeated the beliefs of many major contributors to the golden age of Greece. So revered was he by his followers that he seems to have developed a supernatural aura, which he not only made no attempt to dispel but apparently relished. According to legend embellished in Matthew Arnold's poem "Empedocles on Etna," he died in an attempt to prove his divinity by throwing himself into the mountain's volcanic crater. It would have been difficult to ignore the teachings of a man so determined to prove not only the immortality of his philosophy but of his body as well.

Empedocles's doctrine that all matter is made up of the four elements of fire, air, earth, and water appears to have been the basis on which the concept that—for want of a better term—might be called the principle of fours came into being. To Empedocles, health depended on the harmony of the four elements, since the body, like everything else, is composed of them.

To early physicians, the three visible humors must have needed a fourth in order to conform to the Empedoclean formulation. The mere fact that it was not readily obvious did not stop them. They invented black bile and stretched rather far to justify their belief in its existence, by observations of several "confirmatory" substances: the blackish discharge that sometimes exuded from ulcerated wounds or cancers containing dead tissue; the coffee-grounds character of the vomit brought up by some patients when very sick or near death; the black stool of a person bleeding slowly from the stomach or intestinal tract. It was to these latter two manifestations of critical disease that the Hippocratic aphorism of the early appearance of black bile in stool or vomitus being "a fatal symptom" applies.

As the centuries passed, black bile seems to have become associated with the purplish color of the spleen. By the time Galen codified his concepts in the second century C.E., several groupings of fours had been available for a half millennium, to explain health, disease, and even behavior. As noted in chapter 2, they are the four elements, the four qualities, the four humors, the four sets of characteristics, and the four sources. All of this seemed substantiated by the obvious recurrence each year of the four seasons. Phlegm was most in evidence during the winter (wet and cold), blood in the spring (wet and hot), yellow bile in the summer (dry and hot), and black bile in the autumn (dry and cold). As though to confirm the validity of "the principle of fours," it could also be said—and was—that one or another of the humors is prevalent at each of the four phases of life: blood in childhood, yellow bile in youth, black bile in adulthood, and phlegm in old age.

Not only the Hippocratic school of physicians but all those they would later influence believed these formulations to be useful at the bedsides of the sick. Season, age of patient, climatic conditions, and surroundings could be factored into decisions about how best to keep the humors in balance, using such measures to affect the quantity of each of them as alterations in diet, area of residence, lifestyle changes, purging, puking, bleeding, or botanical preparations. This entire equipage of healing was a self-contained system of medical theory and clinical care, all based on the Empedoclean principle of fours.

But of course, the whole construct depended on the existence of black bile, which had to be fabricated in order to make the theoretical four-part machinery of medicine work. And the symmetry of the system demanded that the hypothetical humor be linked with some organ, as were the three others. Clearly, it would seem to an observer of the classical period, the spleen must be an important structure. In an area where malaria was endemic and splenomegaly therefore frequent, so many people had greatly enlarged spleens that the organ protruding through the abdominal wall was a common sight. Even the liver was often not as easy to feel when a physician put his hand on the belly. Such a substantial structure must surely have a substantial role in the body's functioning. And so, what more worthy organ for the purpose of association with black bile than the spleen, so dark in color and so filled with mystery? Even the reason for its location was a mystery, as was, of course, its very *raison d'être.*

Galen had an answer for everything. He explained the spleen's position by the fabricated fantasy that Nature would have preferred placing it just under the liver so that it might more easily receive that organ's effluvia. But there was a problem. "No available space, however, remained in that region, which was entirely occupied by the stomach, and since there was plenty of room on the left, she placed the spleen there." There was no end to his flights of inventiveness, just as there was no end to the credulousness of physicians for centuries after.

The same is certainly true of the confabulation that black bile causes sadness and depression. Perhaps its supposed acid nature is the reason for the gloom it was said to bring, but there does not otherwise seem any obvious linkage, unless it is the funereal color of the organ that both produces it and oversees its cleansing from the body. The modern mind may be able to understand how characteristics were assigned to blood and phlegm at least, and there may be a tenuous association in the case of yellow bile: blood being the source of life, it was thought to make people lively; a person pouring phlegm out of his nose or coughing it up in huge globs is likely to be subdued and phlegmatic; the association of yellow bile may have been made because many jaundiced people developed personality changes that included irrationality and anger, although this is questionable at best. But far beyond even such a stretch was the construct that a fictional black fluid was responsible for melancholy.

Where might such a far-fetched idea have come from? Perhaps some of the answer can be found in misinterpreted observations of disease. Before autopsies became common in the late eighteenth century, the only malignancies that could be observed were located on the body surface or near the openings of the intestinal and reproductive tracts, where they frequently drained dark material—interpreted as black bile—when ulcerated or decayed. For this reason, these malignancies were believed to be initiated by the body's inability to rid itself of that noxious humor. Throughout the ancient period and well beyond it, an excess of black bile was thought to cause cancer. Accordingly, in addition to the generally lugubrious associations of black bile's impure nature and the foreboding character of its somber-colored organ of supposed origin, the melancholy that is a frequent accompaniment of advanced cancer must have seemed an obvious connection. The melancholy was thought to cause the cancer, instead of the other way around.

(Studies done during the past thirty-five years do present thought-provoking evidence that at least some malignancies and other diseases may indeed be preceded in certain patients by periods of depression, loss, or other kinds of personal upheaval. Though the relationship remains unclear, it has been suggested that one's emotional state plays a far greater role in the genesis of disease than has been heretofore appreciated. In fact, there can be little doubt that certain individuals appear predisposed by traits of personality to be at increased risk of certain illnesses at certain junctures in their lives. But this is a far cry from indicting melancholy as the cause of cancer. No matter how far research eventually goes in studying the psychological context in which disease originates, there will always be far more people depressed by sickness than made sick by depression. Though the Greeks may have been inadvertently prescient in considering the role of emotions, they did so for the wrong reasons. In any event, they badly overplayed their hand—they had their disease theory backward.)

This tendency to put the cart before the horse has plagued medical thought throughout history, and there is no reason to believe that mankind will ever be rid of it. Critical thinking is an approach to observation that has not come easily to the mind of *Homo sapiens,* whether ancient or modern. It sits uncomfortably even today, amidst our more natural and tradition-bound tendency to do otherwise. It takes training, discipline, and a conscious act of will to think analytically, and even then we slip into more accustomed patterns much more readily than we realize.

As we have seen, even a careful observer like van Helmont suffered serious lapses into non sequitur reasoning, which muddled the clarity of his interpretations and led him off into directions far removed from science. As with his conceptions of the stomach, he would take quite a different—and much more exalted—view than did his contemporaries or the ancients of the spleen's effect on the emotions. Because he believed that it provides the acid which he had shown to be crucial to the process of gastric digestion (thereby combining scientific reasoning with pure imagination), he partnered the dark organ with the stomach. To him, the stomach was the shrine wherein dwelt the archeus of the entire person, but the spleen is a participant in the archeus's functions. The spleen, he asserted, sends impulses to the brain, which permit imagination, action, and psychic activity. Although he considered the spleen to be the ultimate origin of emotions and passions, he adamantly denied that it was the origin of melancholy. Quite the opposite. Reasoning that (*a*) many of the mind's activities are determined by messages from the spleen because the archeus dwells in its vicinity, and (*b*) the archeus receives the heavenly light bringing bliss, joy, and happiness, van Helmont declared that the spleen must obviously be the source of smiling and laughter. What a switch from melancholy!

In invoking the notion that some historians have called the smiling spleen, van Helmont was reaching almost as far back into antiquity as did those who believed in its role as the source of black bile and melancholy. Several Roman authors, in fact, refer to the organ as the source of laughter. The satiric poet Persius, writing about 60 C.E., introduced a character who is said to be *sum petulante splene cachinno*, "laughing by virtue of a wanton spleen," but the notion must have existed long before his time. In his *Natural History*, completed in 77 C.E., Pliny the Elder associated intemperance and laughter with a large spleen, as does his contemporary Quintus Serenus Samonicus. According to Serenus, the tendency to inappropriate laughter disappears when the organ is removed, to be replaced by a dour countenance. How he could have known this is beyond guessing, since the likelihood of anyone surviving a splenectomy then must have been tiny or nonexistent.

The Talmudic tractate *Berachoth* also states that the spleen is the source of laughter, but does not further explain itself. The matter was elucidated for Jewish readers around 1100 C.E. by the Spanish rabbinic physician and poet Judah Halevi, who attributed this quality to the spleen's ability to cleanse black bile; when the black bile was gone, happiness and laughter were the result. In the section of the Talmud called the *Mishna Derech Eretz Zuta*, which discusses the microcosm of the body, the spleen is said to regulate the body as the laws of the world regulate the macrocosm. Such an idea, of course, is remarkably close to van Helmont's Christian proposition about the regulating influence of the archeus.

Although as a minor theme, splenic laughter accompanied its more substantially accepted opposite, splenic melancholy, from the Roman period through the Middle Ages and well into the age of science. The laughter tradition seems to have persisted at a rather quiet level until van Helmont revived it with a loud trumpeting of acclamation.

Whatever may have been van Helmont's misconceptions about the spleen, he took a forceful position that began the process by which the thesis of the four humors was eventually destroyed. He pointed out a salient truth that might have been recognized a thousand years earlier had not the stifling hold of Galen's authority prevented it: There is no such thing as black bile. This, he correctly asserted, was reason enough to abandon not only the humoral concept but the entire Galenic explanation of the body's activities. Black bile was the emperor's clothing of medicine.

Van Helmont's timing was perfect. Not only were his writings widely read by the small emerging cadre of scientists during the seventeenth century, but, following closely on the heels of William Harvey's 1628 publication describing the circulation of the blood, they became, like Harvey's book, a great stimulus to studies of human biology. It was no coincidence, for example, that the experiment of animal splenectomy was introduced about this time by the English physician George Thomson, a van Helmont disciple. The operation rapidly became popular not only as a means of studying splenic structure but also in making observations about its function and relationship to the animal's health. In spite of his mysticism, his errors, and even his certainty of the smiling spleen, van Helmont is a hero who deserves to be less unsung than he is.

The notion that the spleen is the source not only of melancholy but of laughter too is incorporated into its definition in Samuel Johnson's dictionary of 1755 as is yet another symptom of moodiness: anger. In the statement that the organ "is supposed the seat of anger, melancholy and mirth," Johnson's usage was that of the general public of the time. But by then, the notion had arisen over the course of several centuries that there exists a specific clinical condition called Spleen, diagnosable by physicians and compatible within the general pattern we nowadays call depression.

Even among the laity, the major splenic theme was melancholy, although this had somehow become mixed with peevishness and anger sometime after the sixteenth century, and sometimes also with morbid preoccupation concerning imagined illness. The world's literature, particularly in English, has been enriched by the many volumes of poetry and prose devoted to the condition that gradually came to be called Spleen and its generalized symptoms, such as gloom, sullenness, wrath, and hypochondria. The names of Pope, Swift, Sterne, and Byron come up repeatedly when such literary productions are discussed, as do those of less well known English writers such as Matthew Green, Anne Finch, Elizabeth Carter, and Edward Young. In another country and another time, few modern readers can think of the condition called Spleen without it bringing to mind the unfinished collection of prose poems by Charles Baudelaire, *Le Spleen de Paris.*

In 1621, the Anglican clergyman Robert Burton published an entire seven hundred forty–page book devoted to the condition. Entitled *Anatomy of Melancholy,* the text is preceded by a poem of forty-eight couplets, described as "The Author's Abstract of Melancholy," the six final lines of which will suffice to illustrate the state of mind of people afflicted with an extreme case of Spleen. Anyone who has suffered the anguish of clinical depression will understand these three couplets:

> My pain's past cure, another hell,
> I may not in this torment dwell!
> Now desperate, I hate my life,
> Lend me a halter [hangman's noose] or a knife;
> > All my griefs to this are folly,
> > Naught so damn'd as melancholy.

Of the many similar descriptions of the condition appearing during this time, a particularly poignant one is to be found at the conclusion of an ode written about 1694, shortly after its author had recovered from a serious bout of depression. In "The Spleen," Anne Finch, later to be Countess of Winchilsea, addressed herself directly to the disease, decrying not only its excruciating symptoms but its inscrutable and protean nature, presenting as panic, gloom, insomnia, and delusional thinking, all at once and separately. Even physicians, she laments, are not able to find its source:

> Or, through the well-dissected body trace
> The secret, the mysterious ways,
> By which thou dost surprise, and prey upon the mind.

Near the end of her ode, Finch speaks of the famed Dr. Richard Lower, not only a pioneer in experimental blood transfusion and in studies of the heart but also London's most prominent physician of the period. Like some others of his colleagues, Lower believed he might learn about melancholy the same way he was accustomed to studying other diseases—by dissection of the human cadaver. Addressing the disease itself, Finch describes the tragic outcome of the doctor's obsessional pursuit of a source, whether it might prove to be in the spleen or elsewhere:

> Though in the search, too deep for human thought,
> With unsuccessful toil he wrought,
> Till thinking thee to've catched, himself by thee caught,
> Retained thy prisoner, thy acknowledged slave,
> And sank beneath thy chain to a lamented grave.

The public recognition accorded to *Anatomy of Melancholy* reflected the wide contemporary prevalence of the condition called Spleen, and the frequency with which it was discussed in the literature, the parlor, and everyday discourse, not to say the doctor's consulting room. Between those who had it, those who imagined it, and those who aspired to it because it was thought to confer a certain aesthetic superiority on its sufferers, the condition was so common in Great Britain that many thought of it as a particularly English problem. In 1713 Joseph Addison had referred to this phenomenon in the pages of the *Spectator:* "Melancholy is a kind of demon that haunts our island, and often conveys herself to us in an easterly wind."

Not only was melancholy—Spleen—thought to be an especially English condition but *most* especially a condition of the favored classes of society. In 1733, the prominent English physician George Cheyne wrote a book about nervous diseases in general and those related to Spleen in particular, which he chose to entitle *The English Malady,* because continental Europeans had given that name to the syndrome: "The Title I have chosen for this Treatise, is a Reproach universally thrown on this Island by Foreigners, and all our Neighbors on the Continent, by whom nervous Distempers, Spleen, Vapours, and Lowness of Spirits, are in Derision, called the ENGLISH MALADY."

In his preface, Cheyne agrees with those foreigners, and lists climatic, dietary, and cultural reasons why the continental detractors are correct, including "the Inactivity and sedentary Occupations of the better Sort (among whom this Evil mostly rages) . . . These nervous disorders being computed to make almost one third of the Complaints of the People of Condition in England." Spleen was thus not just an English ailment per se, but a fashionable one too. To be afflicted with it was to be of a kind with those of substance and refinement, the "People of Condition."

Eight years before Cheyne's publication, Sir Richard Blackmore, a skilled physician and failed writer of poems ("dreadful" would have been more accurate; even his obituary called him "an eminent physician but a very indifferent poet") combined his medical and literary interests in writing *A Treatise of the Spleen and Vapours or Hypochondriacal and Hysterical Affections.* As did so many other commentators of the time, Blackmore blended together, in his subtitle, two mood disorders: hypochondriacal problems caused by the spleen and hysterical ones (commonly called The Vapours) traditionally related to the uterus. As he put it, "[T]he primitive practitioners ascribed Hysterical Passions to noxious Fumes and Vapours, ascending I know not how, from the Womb."

Though he felt free to range all over the intellectual lot in his discussion of splenic function and its effect on mood, Blackmore began his discourse with a confession that accurately describes the real state of knowledge of the spleen at the time:

[N]otwithstanding all the Improvements and Advances hitherto made by Anatomists and Physicians, an immense Number of

Difficulties are still behind, which the most sagacious and accomplished Wits are altogether incapable of unriddling.

The use of this considerable Bowel [a general term, used at the time to refer to any abdominal organ] is one of the numerous Classes of Phaenomena, that remain unexplained. It has eluded the Searches of the tracing [dissecting] Knife, and the acutest Reason, and continues the Reproach of Anatomists, and the Dishonour of Physicians, while Multitudes of the most eminent Sons of the Art have attempted to disclose this great Secret in vain, so that the Capacities of Men have hitherto proven unequal to the difficult Task.

Of course, this disclosure did not prevent Blackmore from furthering a reputation he had long-since acquired for gassy pomposity, by pontificating for the three hundred following pages on the real functions of the spleen as he saw them. As to melancholia, hypochondriasis, and the like, he was, as were so many others, convinced that these emotions cause swelling of both spleen and liver but, "I must declare, that in my Judgment, what we call the Spleen, is a Distemper belonging to the whole System of the Animal Spirits, and has its Rise immediately from Them." In other words, Spleen may cause the spleen to swell (an imaginary finding, but one nevertheless sworn to by virtually every physician of the time), but its real cause is the buildup in that organ, and in the liver too, of a vitalistic quality known in those days as animal spirits, coming from all the organs of the body.*

Blackmore was further convinced that the spleen has no purpose to the individual, a notion that had originally been promulgated in the third century B.C.E. by the Greek physiologist Erasistratus but largely

---

*The Greek-derived term for "under the ribs" is hypochondrium, whose adjective in English is hypochondriac. Because the spleen lies under the lower ribs (as does the liver, on the other side), symptoms thought to originate in it or affecting either spleen or liver or both are said to be hypochondriac. The term has been used since the classical period to signify complaints that seem to have no cause. All of this is complicated by another factor, which was the ancient belief that the uterus leaps about in the abdominal cavity. A woman can develop hypochondriacal symptoms if her womb rises up to a hypochondriac position.

ignored in subsequent centuries. Blackmore based his opinions on the fact that he was unable to identify any demonstrable effect on the bodies of animals in which the organ had been removed. But as a firm adherent of the Galenic doctrine that nature creates no structure without a function, he argued that if the spleen has no usefulness for the individual, then "it must be of some important Use for the Continuation of the Species." It was, after all, "a Bowel of such Distinction in the Body, of such a Magnitude, such an artful Composition, and endowed with such numerous Vessels" that there would seem no question that it was designed by nature for some purpose of great significance. That significance, he assured his readers, was "some remote yet considerable Office, by which it promotes the Propagation of the Species." In other words, the spleen, in some remote way, participates in reproduction. Needless to say, Blackmore failed to tell just how that was accomplished.

But, like all his countrymen, Blackmore was certain that the high prevalence of Spleen was evidence of British superiority over all other nationalities:

> But of all these different People, the Temper of the Natives of *Britain* [italics in original] is most various, which proceeds from the Spleen, an ingredient of their Constitution, which is almost peculiar, at least in the Degree of it, to this Island. Hence arises the Diversity of Genius and Disposition, of which this Soil is so fertile.

And so, a silver lining glistened within the dark cloud of Spleen's gloom, at least for Englishmen. Spleen was not only fashionable, but it conferred an intellectual and moral superiority that confirmed the uniqueness of "People of Condition" of the sceptered isle. Ignored or forgotten was melancholy's frequency in every class of society and every nation. Others may not have indulged themselves in it quite so much as a prosperous or intellectual Briton, but clinical depression, which is the factor uniting so many of the symptoms of Spleen, is hardly the property of any national or social group.

But whatever erroneous ideas he may have cherished about the spleen's function, Blackmore did recognize that the impressive structure he had spent so many years studying must exist for reasons so significant that even he was unable to divine them:

> It is impossible to inspect and contemplate this large Organ, without concluding, that it must have some important Office in the Animal Administration and that this is not a superfluous and impertinent Fungus, or an Error or Sport of Nature.

Blackmore and others had plenty of opportunity to "inspect and contemplate this large Organ" because, following on George Thomson's introduction of the procedure, animal splenectomy had become a standard experiment by the middle of the seventeenth century. Not only had such operations proven that a splenectomized creature could survive, but they had provided plenty of organs to study, with both the naked eye and the microscope. In 1666, the Italian anatomist Marcello Malpighi had identified distinctive nodules on the spleen's cut surface, which he at first thought to be glands. Two centuries later, they would be recognized as collections of white blood cells clustered around a tiny central artery. To this day, they are called Malpighian bodies.

At the time Blackmore was writing about the spleen's "important Office," some inkling of what that office might be had already been put forth by a highly respected London physician, William Stukeley. When Stukeley was honored by the invitation of the Royal College of Physicians to present the annual Goulstonian Lecture in 1722, he chose as his topic "The Spleen: Its Description and History," using that illustrious forum to debunk—as would Blackmore three years later—some of the time-honored erroneous notions of splenic function and a few of those that had recently appeared. Among the latter was the Malpighi-inspired belief that the spleen contained glands which secrete various juices. Stukeley, convinced of his observation that splenectomized dogs "become more gay and brisk than before, and swifter in running," introduced a few other ill-conceived ideas. Nevertheless, he did correctly recognize that, "I see nothing but what seems to confirm my position of the spleen being an animal sponge, not a gland to separate juice, but a receptacle of pure and good blood for great and wise ends in Nature." What Stukeley had done was to convert the ancient doctrine of purification into a contemporary model that recognized, thanks to Harvey's discovery, the vast volume of blood that circulated through the organ and the probability that blood might contain contaminants of which it had to be purged.

And so, Stukeley was ahead of his contemporaries in conceiving of the spleen as a sort of sponge. As it turned out, the human spleen would be found to function not so much as a "receptacle" (although it does perform that reservoir function in the dogs used in his experiments) as it would a guarantor that the blood would be maintained in "pure and good" condition.

Real understanding of splenic function developed slowly and did not achieve a strongly scientific basis until shortly after the beginning of the nineteenth century. But even slower was the disappearance of the belief that the spleen affects the state of emotions. People in general and the English in particular clung to the fancy as though to a part of their identity, which in a sense it was. Even after it had become generally known to have no basis in fact, by the middle of the nineteenth century, the notion continued to exist so vividly in language that we occasionally turn to it today as though it has real meaning. Very likely, there are those who still believe that it does.

The improved microscopes that became available in the 1830s allowed for more meticulous anatomical observations than had previously been possible, and the rapid growth of biochemistry and physiology later in the century added much new information. A great deal of progress was stimulated by the general acceptance of the germ theory in the 1880s, but it was not really until the very modern era of immunological sophistication of approximately the past thirty years that the full range of the spleen's many functions was appreciated. Even during my medical school days in the 1950s there was still plenty of reason to invoke Galen's pronouncement, *plenum mysterii organum.* Ergo, the Winternitz story.

Today we know that the human spleen has two major varieties of function. In its "sponge" role, it acts as a filter; in its immunologic role, it takes part in many processes that enable the body to resist infection.

It would in time be discovered that blood circulates through the spleen in two ways, fast and slow. In general the fast circulation serves the purposes of the organ's nutrition, just as in any other structure of the body. The slow circulation allows the blood to meander through the organ's pulpy substance, where damaged or ineffective cells are removed, as are bacteria and various forms of microscopic debris. In addition, the spleen as sponge excises certain superfluous structures within blood cells without destroying the cells themselves. The spleen's immunologic functions are many and varied, but can best be summarized by the brief statement that it is the site where immune responses are produced against blood-borne foreign substances called antigens.

Because of the developing spleen's antibacterial and other immunologic functions, its removal when a patient is young can cause difficulties in fighting infection. This problem was not generally recognized until first reported in 1952. By the early 1970s, the emerging evidence had persuaded pediatricians and surgeons that all possible attempts should be made to preserve some part of the spleen, however small, when injury or other pathology required that the organ be excised. Not only is great care taken to avoid splenectomy nowadays, but numerous methods have been developed to leave at least a bit of functioning tissue intact when surgery cannot be avoided.

But even with all we now know about the spleen, some mystery still remains. Without doubt, the next few decades will witness splenic discoveries that are today unpredictable, and we will learn of even more vital roles played in our moment-to-moment lives by the organ that Erasistratus thought had no function.

But about one function, there can be no doubt: Removing the spleen has never made anyone a fast runner. The unfulfilled Sherwins of the world will have to seek their salvation elsewhere. Jim Bornemann did not become a speedier soccer player after being separated from his spleen. And even were I really and truly willing to give up mine, I would afterward continue to galumph along just as slowly and clumsily as I do today.

CHAPTER SEVEN

THE HEART:

CRACKING

THE VALVE

So the heart is the beginning of life, the Sun of the Microcosm, even as the Sun deserves to be call'd the heart of the world; for it is the heart by whose virtue and pulsation the blood is moved, perfected, made apt to nourish, and is preserved from corruption and coagulation; it is the household divinity which, discharging its function, nourishes, cherishes, quickens the whole body, and is indeed the foundation of life, the source of all action.

WILLIAM HARVEY, 1628
On the Motion of the Heart and Blood in Animals, Chapter VIII

ARVEY might have added that the heartbeat is the background rhythm to which we live our lives. It is the cadence within our days, the predictable essence that will be unchanged tomorrow from today and from all our yesterdays. It ends only when we end. The heart's metronomic regularity is the reassuring signal for which our deepest selves unknowingly listen, the message of continuity and the pulsing presence proclaiming the certainty that we endure. In the ancient formulation of macrocosm and microcosm, the heart is the sun.

The life of each of our seventy-five trillion cells depends on the uninterrupted beat of the heart, and in more ways than we can consciously know, so does the inner perception that we are in harmony with all that surrounds us. Though your or my distinctive pulsing source is unique, awareness of it makes each of us at one with all living things. The heartbeat unites us to one another even as it separates us. Every man thus marches to his own drummer—every woman treads a measure that is hers alone. And yet we share the heart's throbbing euphony. It regulates the course of humankind's journey through the days of our years.

The heart has fascinated me since the very first time I saw its forceful scarlet thrusting within the opened chest of an anesthetized laboratory animal almost fifty years ago. It seemed at that instant ready to leap out at me with each rising, clenching beat—were it not for the fibrous folds of tissue holding it securely in place, it might very well have done precisely that. The compact red generator of life was bursting, I thought, with far too much energy to remain long confined within the firm enclosure of the animal's rib cage. It appeared at any second about to propel its way upward to the ceiling of that room. And yet, explosive with barely restrained power as it obviously was, there seemed nevertheless a kind of assured serenity in the heart's continuing repetition of the alternating clench-and-relax rhythm, hundreds of dependable, uniform times during the several minutes I stood there transfixed before it. Though I would certainly have denied it at that chemistry-and-physics-dominated period of my life, I watched that rabbit's heart with a sense of awe.

I have never lost that awe. It remains with me in spite of all I have since learned of the heart's nuts and bolts and valves and cords—not to mention its flows and its fluid forces, its electricity and its chemical influences. I know them and know also the heart's weaknesses just as well as I do any other part of this human body of ours that I have never stopped studying since those youthful days. And yet, the thorough familiarity with cardiac anatomy and physiology—and romance and breakability—has not lessened by an iota the spell cast on me when I first gazed at it that day in the laboratory.

Very early, I turned my fascination with the heart to practical use. Ever since its founding in 1810, my medical school has required that a research study be done and a doctoral thesis be written by all candidates for the M.D. degree. Intrigued as I was with the marvels of cardiac performance to which I was being repeatedly exposed, I knew immediately my choice of topic—I would study the heart. Having in college become interested in the electrical accompaniments of biological processes, I selected as my thesis adviser a cardiologist whose field of research was the elucidation of the electrocardiogram's sources. That felicitous choice had the added advantage that the professor allowed me to accompany him when he occasionally did late-evening consultations at a small community hospital about fifteen miles down the shoreline from New Haven. The hospital being inadequately equipped, even for 1952, it was my job to carry the unwieldy portable EKG machine from my mentor's car to the room of the patient being evaluated. It was a quid pro quo: In return for hauling the EKG machine, I was granted the incomparable privilege of hauling The Great Man's EKG Machine. I thought it a major honor, and so did he.

Together, he and I—but mostly he—devised an experiment in which I stimulated the main pumping chamber, the left ventricle, of a dog's heart to contract whenever I set it off with a small current. The idea was to study the electrical field produced during the so-called ectopic (meaning "not in the normal place") beat caused by the stimulus. This required that I operate on each of the dogs I planned to study, in order to stitch one end of a specially prepared wire called an electrode onto the surface of the ventricle and lead its other end out through the chest wall so that I could hook it up to a source of current. The purpose of these experiments was to obtain valuable information about the propagation of the electrical wave that activates the normal heart.

I would begin a typical experiment early on the morning of the appointed day, performing the surgery, stitching up the dog's chest, and allowing the animal to recover for a few hours while being kept lightly anesthetized. I then spent the afternoon and usually much of the evening stimulating the sleeping animal's heart repeatedly, by firing a burst of current over and over again through the wire, as I moved a monitoring probe from one to another of a hundred or so points I had previously marked out on the clean-shaven chest wall. At every location, I would take a measurement during an individual ectopic beat, patiently moving the tiny probe on to the next point and then shocking the heart again, until the voltage generated by the beat had been noted at every one of the many spots and recorded on EKG paper. Looking back on the strange experiment, it seems a wonder that I never killed a dog or myself during the multitudes of firings and simultaneous determinations.

The whole tedious process felt like it took forever. No matter my sense of accomplishment at the final results of each laborious experiment, the dreary road to its completion was cheerless and exquisitely boring. Having not yet experienced the epiphany that would later make a surgeon of me, I hated the operations and resented the mindless repetition of firing one shock after another—and concomitantly taking one measurement after another—for hours on end. It didn't help that the dogs were provided by a city pound where they had been penned up for at least a month until the authorities could be sure they would not be claimed by distressed owners. They were greasy and dirty; shaving them did not help much. Not only was the smell intolerable but the sleeping animals had a disconcerting way of urinating frequently and with great force. Worse yet, they seemed always to spontaneously empty their capacious rectums onto the laboratory table sometime between the sixth and eighth hours of the experiment.

My only consolation was that I shared the misery with my classmate Joseph Ignatius Boylan, Jr., a fellow Bronxite who was using exactly the same animal preparation to study an entirely different phenomenon, albeit one requiring the repeated taking of electrocardiograms. Joe would assist me at the operation and then begin his electrical calculations after I had finished mine. When the whole loathsome extravaganza was completed, we would overdose the dog with intravenous barbiturate. An autopsy of the chest was necessary to be sure that the electrodes had remained in proper position and no damage had been inflicted on the multiply shocked heart. It was our habit to carry out that study right there amid the cloacal pool of feces and urine. At the end of such a disgusting procedure, the real challenge was deciding which to do first: would we go back to our rooming houses and take a prolonged shower using antiseptic soap, or would we just give in to the powerful urge to fall exhausted into bed?

Joe and I marked the EKG paper each time an individual determination was made so that we could have a record of the point where it had been taken. The paper was allowed to spew out of the machine and onto the floor, to be rolled up at the end of the entire experiment for later study. From time to time, we would have to pause to replace a completed roll, but we otherwise made no attempt to maintain any degree of neatness, since it would have only prolonged the time we had to spend with the foul-smelling dog. When we had completed an experiment, the laboratory floor would be covered with endless coils of the ribbonlike paper, which we would then roll up and analyze at our leisure on some future day.

I remember as though it were yesterday one experiment on a very big dog in which either Joe or I or both required an unusually large number of determinations, with the result that we did not finish our work until an hour after dawn on the day following the surgery. Needless to say, we were at least knee-deep in curlicues of EKG paper by the time we had done Joe's final tracing, at approximately 7:00 A.M. As we gazed in dismay at the hundreds of yards of twisted convolutions covering the entire floor of the small laboratory, the door unexpectedly opened and Jake the janitor (known to our entire class of medical students by his honorific, Jake the Janitor) appeared, to do his early-morning cleanup before the staff arrived to begin work. He took one startled look at the dead and hairless hound lying flat on its back in a puddle of its own filth—all four legs pointing upward in different directions—and then fixed his appalled gaze on the two grim-faced, bleary-eyed, unshaven young men staring wearily back at him. Only after regarding us in this bewildered way for a few seconds did his eyes drop to the endless spirals of cluttered EKG paper in which we stood surrounded almost up to our mid-thighs. Aghast, he appeared unable to take in the whole scene at once, and began to twist his head now toward one of the sickening sights and then toward another, in complete disbelief. After a few turns at this, he suddenly exclaimed "Oh shit—NO!" and slammed the door shut again, no doubt to expunge the entire horrible apparition from his field of vision. We could hear him clumsily thudding his acutely crazed way down the hall, obviously in a state of panic that he might have to return later and clean up the indescribable mess.

Open to its acknowledgments page, the doctoral dissertation that resulted from my prolonged anguish—euphoniously entitled *Field Functions of a Forced Ventricular Extrasystole*—is lying alongside my arm as I write about those long-ago events. In the section's final paragraph, I thank my "classmate and friend, Mr. Joseph Boylan, for many weary hours, both day and night, of what must have been the most tiresome, uninspiring labor, and most of all for his never-failing good nature." Those grueling experiments were the only "tiresome, uninspiring" experience I ever had with the heart during my medical school days or at any other time. Almost always, I was thrilled to be in its presence, where I had some of the most engrossing moments of the early part of my career.

Among them was the first time I took part in an operation on a human heart. I was a third-year student newly assigned to the cardiac surgery service, whose chief was a man I'll call Dr. James Jackson Wiggins Brock, a soft-spoken but nevertheless extremely intense South Carolinian then in the early phases of the most productive years of what would be a distinguished career. Dr. Brock's gentle drawl belied a compulsive attention to even the minutest detail of each operative procedure. So demanding was he in his meticulousness that an operation took two or three times longer in his hands than it might when done by most other surgeons. The extra hours were spent satisfying his insistent thoroughness and almost obsessional determination to do things in the safest possible manner.

As maddening as it was to his assistants, the methodical exactitude of Brock's technique paid large dividends. In those days before open

heart surgery and high-tech anesthesia, he had accumulated an envi-
able record of success, with extremely low rates of mortality and complications. For certain of the operations done at that time, in fact, an
approach that to others seemed unnecessarily finicky and even timid
was the reason that no one in the country had a higher success rate
than he did.

Unlike most surgeons, who placed the medical student either far
down the operating table or awkwardly positioned at the end of one of
the retractors that held the wound open, Brock kept the neophyte at
his right side during the entire procedure. Although one could never
know what was going on in the surgeon's vigilantly focused mind or
perceive the sensation in his sometimes tentative fingertips, the student enjoyed an ideal view of even the smallest detail of each operation. He might be totally enervated by the time the last stitch had been
placed anywhere from five to twelve or more hours after the induction
of anesthesia, but he had seen cardiac surgery from a perspective available to students in few other hospitals.

THE patient was a thirty-one-year-old woman whom I'll call Lily
Stewart (both for confidentiality and because I don't remember her
name), suffering from a condition called mitral stenosis, in those days
and now most commonly encountered years or decades after a childhood or adolescent bout of rheumatic fever. The disease causes scarring and the accumulation of thick fibrous tissue on the edges of the
valve that lies between the reservoirlike left atrium (which receives
oxygenated blood returning from the lungs) and the ventricle below
it (which is the powerful pumping chamber that forces the blood out
to the body). The flexibility of the valve is thus impaired, preventing it
from opening and closing as easily as it should. Not only that, but the
scarring causes adhesions between the two delicate leaflets of tissue
that form the valve, further inhibiting its movements. The result is a
narrowing that partially obstructs the blood flow downward from the
atrium into the ventricle. Some of the blood accordingly backs up into
the lungs, causing congestion and progressive shortness of breath. As

the condition worsens, breathing becomes very difficult and the right side of the heart may weaken and fail in its attempt to push blood through the lungs. The disease is diagnosed by its symptoms and by the presence of a murmur with a characteristic rumble, immediately following a snapping sound caused by the contracting atrium forcing the resistant valve open by pushing a bolus of blood against it.

Mitral stenosis was one of the earliest cardiac diseases to be treated successfully by surgery, in an operation called valvulotomy—literally, opening up the valve. Some ten or a dozen attempts were made in the 1920s with only two surviving patients. The results being so poor, no further such operations were known until the mid 1940s, when several successes, first in Philadelphia and shortly thereafter in Boston and London, were achieved. Following these, the operation soon became standardized, so that by the time I was a student on the wards between 1953 and 1955, many thousands were being done in hospitals throughout the world. With slight variations, two methods were in favor. In one, the valve leaflets were separated by a specially designed knife inserted through the heart wall; in the other, the surgeon cut a small hole in the atrium, just large enough to accept his index finger, which he then lowered into the valve so that he could force it open. Either way, the idea was to free up the fibrous tissue and separate the fused leaflets, in order to allow them to move more freely.

Because Lily Stewart had been in the hospital for a week before she arrived in the operating room, I had had plenty of opportunity to spend time with her and assess her condition. The medical student evaluation of a newly admitted patient takes—or at least took in 1953—about two hours, so that the full history could be heard and a thorough physical examination completed. This alone meant that I knew my patient at least as well as did the other members of the team, and probably better than anyone except Dr. Brock himself.

Mrs. Stewart was a thin, ginger-haired woman who would have appeared pale but for the high flush over her cheekbones and the slight bluish tinge of her lips and earlobes, caused by decreased oxygenation of the blood as it made its difficult way through the crowded circuit of the lungs. Most striking was the shortness of breath, even when she was at rest and sitting up with three pillows behind her head. Removing even one of them worsened her breathing problems, and she found the loss of two unmanageable. During the admission interview, she answered my questions with very short sentences, because respirations became more difficult each time she began to speak. Obviously, her lungs were congested with backed-up blood under high pressure. The breathlessness made her fidgety; she picked at the bedclothes from time to time during our conversation and constantly held her chin high in an attempt to get more air. Speaking to her was like trying to have a conversation with someone who has just crossed the finish line of a marathon.

Mrs. Stewart had recently begun to experience a new symptom that she said was even more alarming to her than the shortness of breath with which she had long been familiar: Several times during our interview, she was seized with an alarming paroxysm of coughing, during which she spat small amounts of bright-red sputum into a Kleenex she held always ready in her hand. The tiny vessels in the lungs were under such high pressure that they were spontaneously rupturing.

Being a very young man, I was much impressed—perhaps sympathetic is a better word—with one of my patient's symptoms that was completely new to me. She had stopped having intercourse with her husband six months earlier because the combination of the emotion and the necessity for at least an element of position-change or recumbency had each time worsened the distress of her air hunger so suddenly that she was invariably thrown into an acute and terrifying episode that felt like she was drowning in the gurgly, pinkish secretions that would begin coming up from her lungs. Actually, it was her husband who told me about this—even had she wanted to, she did not have the breath to string together enough words to relate the entire story.

Over the few days following her admission, my visits to Mrs. Stewart were brief. Not only did her breathing problems preclude all but the most momentary exchanges, but she was quite obviously too exhausted with the effort of respiration for any but those contacts that were absolutely necessary. When she tried to nap she was likely to awaken suddenly after only a few minutes, gasping for the oxygen that made its way only with great difficulty into the swollen blood vessels around the air sacs in her heavy lungs. It was clear that she could not long survive in such a state. Though the risk was great, she was desperate to have the operation.

Lily Stewart was the sort of patient who in those more blunt-spoken times we used to call a cardiac cripple. Even before the rapid worsening that had brought her to this present fearful condition, she could do no housework, was unable to care for her two young children, and rarely went outdoors. Not only had her days become unlivable but there were not many of them left. Her only chance for survival was the high-risk surgery. Just before she was wheeled into the OR suite on the designated morning, she wordlessly gripped her husband's hand and kissed him for what he later told me he was sure would be the last time.

When I arrived at the OR, Mrs. Stewart was sitting up on a gurney outside of room 3. Although her eyes were closed, small, fresh tears rested on her lashes. Hurrying by, I spied Dr. Brock entering the senior surgeons' locker room. As I would later discover was his invariable habit, he had stopped at his patient's side and stood by her for a few moments, speaking gently and doing all that he could to be encouraging. Whatever were the turbulent thoughts that must have been racing through the worried mind of that uncommon man, he would never have conveyed to a patient anything but optimism and quiet reassurance. He could hardly have felt them himself on that portentous morning that we were now embarking upon with such a sense of foreboding. Uncertainty, fretfulness, impatience—those who served as his assistants bore the brunt of his complex bundle of emotional tics, but never did a single patient suspect that their surgeon was anything other than a self-assured icon of solidity.

Like the rest of us, Brock was worried, first of all, about what might happen during the induction of anesthesia. Even in the most skillful of hands, these preliminary manipulations can precipitate a sudden abnormality of rhythm or a worsening of heart failure from which a patient as sick as ours might not be rescuable. But luck was with the anesthesiologist and Mrs. Stewart. The induction was accomplished without untoward event, the breathing tube was slid into her windpipe, and her sleeping body was rotated on the table so that she lay on her right side, ready for the operation to begin. The resident, whom I'll call Fred Clarke, and I took up our positions after the intern had swabbed the chest with antiseptic solution and applied the large drapes so that only a wide swath of its left side was exposed.

With a long sweep of his arm, Fred cut through the skin and underlying skimpy layer of fat, making a gradually curving incision that began alongside the breastbone and ran backward over the chest wall, ending at a point some two inches below the tip of the shoulder blade behind. The muscles he exposed with the cut were some of those well known to bodybuilders—the latissimus dorsi, the serratus anterior, and a bit of the trapezius—but in our patient they were so thin that cutting through them with the scalpel and tying off their blood vessels was the work of only a few minutes. As each of them came into view, I was asked its name and function, questions so routinely put to medical students that I was well prepared for them.

Soon the length of the fourth rib lay exposed before us, like an arching strut protecting the vital organs that pulsed and breathed, expanded and contracted, within the rigidly encased cavity of the chest. Using a set of scraperlike tools, Fred peeled away the rib's fibrous covering, finally detaching the bone from the deep muscles that lay between it and the ribs just higher and lower, numbers three and five. Once the rib was stripped of its thin cover, it was a simple matter to divide its attachment to the cartilage in front and then cut across its narrow width far back among the vertical muscles running up and down alongside the spinal column. Fred lifted the rib out of its snug cradle and cut through the pleura, that final filmy layer lining the inside of the chest cavity.

The first thing I saw as the pleura fell away under Fred's scalpel was the spongy pinkness of the underlying lung, sliding up and down under the incision as the breathing machine forced anesthetic gas and oxygen into it and then allowed the exhaled mixture to escape. More than the usual pressure was being required to expand its turgid texture, but I did not know that at the time. To me, the salmon-coral color, the smooth gliding motion of the great lobed organ under the pleura, the certainty that I was about to see the heart—all of it was exhilarating.

A double-bladed spreading retractor was now put into place and ratcheted up in the gap where the fourth rib had been. The motion forced ribs three and five widely apart and made the long narrow opening in the chest wall big enough to easily accept the insertion of two pairs of hands, various instruments, and a few large cloth pads moistened with warm saline solution. The pads were spread out over the lung, and the entire package gently drawn backward out of the way, exposing the sturdy fibrous envelope called the pericardium, through which the powerful pulsations of the contained heart could now be seen.

Until this point, conversation had been continuous, but focused only on the job at hand. The word that had been used to describe Lily Stewart's condition was *precarious,* and her operation was not one to be approached with anything but extreme gravity. Fred, in most circumstances a cheerful fellow whose easy banter kept the members of his team distracted from the serious tasks before them, was uncharacteristically subdued that morning. Perhaps he was identifying with the young husband, a man about his own age waiting anxiously outside the OR, the future of his family and of his life hanging by tenuous threads on the events unfolding on that operating table. Or the resident may simply have been concerned with the probability that his chief would be even more demanding—or worse yet, unreasonable—than usual on that particularly nerve-wracking day, when any small mishap might be lethal to a young woman already so close to death.

The relationship between Fred Clarke and the chief was complex. Like most of our residents in those days, Fred had matured in the crucible of overseas service in World War II. At thirty-nine, Brock was only about five years older than his resident, and though far more experienced at surgery, he had enormous respect for the younger man's dependability and judgment. It was clear that he saw Fred more as a supportive and confident younger brother than a trainee. The two spoke to each other almost as equals. It was well known among the students that when feeling less than sure of himself, Brock depended on Fred's reassuring presence to steady him. But there was never any doubt about who the boss was.

So intent on our work had the entire team been that no one noticed the surgeon enter from the scrub room, water dripping from his upraised forearms and ready to be gowned. When Brock was completely outfitted in the surgeon's sterile regalia, we repositioned ourselves around the table.

I took up my place alongside and up-table of him, our bodies touching from shoulder to knee. I had been warned that he would be hesitant, uncertain, and particularly irritable when doing such a hazardous operation, but he seemed remarkably sure of himself and decisive as he took over command from Fred. Apprehensive as I was— it was my first cardiac operation and the patient was desperately ill—I felt reassured by the warmth of the chief's body next to mine. He had a few words with the anesthesiologist and Fred about the patient's status, asked me a question or two about cardiac physiology, and got right down to work.

The very first thing Brock did was to make a long up-and-down slit in the pericardium. He peeled its edges back out of the way and exposed the living, beating heart. Though it may have appeared flabby and sick to every other person in that room, the fist-sized dynamo of thrusting power which just then seemed to fill my entire field of vision was a sight so unprecedented in its glorious fulfillment that I felt as though I had been waiting to see it since the day I was born.

For here was indeed the beginning of life, the sun of the microcosm, and as far as I was concerned it was at that moment more brilliant than the sun of the *mac*rocosm. It was my own household divinity—nourishing, cherishing, quickening my whole body as I stared at it. It was the source of all action, of all energy, of all the driving force that a human being possesses. I was dumbstruck in its presence, so distracted by the ineffable beauty of the thing that I let my fingers loosen from the flat, ribbonlike retractor I had been given to hold the lung out of the way with. I was jerked back to reality by

Brock's instant outburst of displeasure, although in fact the brief sample of his legendary temper was mild: "C'mon, son, wake up. This little lady needs you to pay attention to her!"

The problem, of course, was not that I had been asleep, but quite the opposite: something in me had been awakened. I stood there in a heightened state of awareness, all of it focused on the magnificence before me and none of it on my assigned task. Brock's admonition broke—or at least weakened—the spell. My rapt absorption receded just enough to disperse the drifting thoughts and return me to the company of the operating team.

In continuity with the side of the atrium is its antechamber—the auricle—a flattened appendage lying against it much as an ear does alongside the head. It is as though nature designed the auricle for the benefit of the cardiac surgeon. Because it is essentially a cul-de-sac off the atrium, it allows him to enter that reservoir unobtrusively. This is what Brock now proceeded to do.

Having placed a specially designed clamp across the auricle and inserted a series of anchoring stitches, he cut a slit into its wall just large enough to admit his right index finger. As he carried out these maneuvers, Lily Stewart's hypersensitive heart demonstrated just how easily it could become agitated, breaking into an alarming shower of irregular beats. With this, the blood pressure dropped about 20 millimeters of mercury, but only until the irregularity spontaneously abated after Brock stopped the forward motion of his finger. With a heart that is so easily upset, it behooves the surgeon to move with extra caution, and Brock's usual deliberate slowness became a circumspect crawl.

With utmost care, the surgeon began again to advance his finger into the auricle and announced that he was moving it gradually through the atrium and down toward the diseased valve. Watching that finger disappearing bit by bit into the depths of the heart, I tried to visualize the scene within, as the disembodied digit made its silent way through the streaming blood, coming ever closer to its fateful destination. The perilous journey was interrupted several times by brief runs of irregular beats. Finally, after what seemed an hour but must

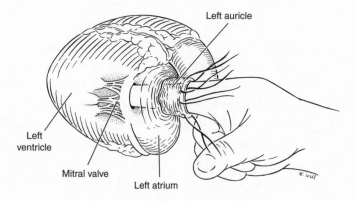

Diagram of mitral valvulotomy. The surgeon's finger is projecting through the atrium and entering the valve.

have been only a few minutes, Glenn announced that he was positioned just above the valve and was preparing to enter it.

It was part of Brock's scrupulously organized protocol at this point in the operation to call out the numbers "1, 2, 3!" to let the operating team and the anesthesiologist know that he was set to enter the valve itself. The purpose of the signaling was to alert all warriors that the battle was about to begin in earnest and everyone had better be prepared for any untoward eventuality, be it rhythm disturbances, hemorrhage, or even cardiac arrest. He was the man whose surgical motto was "An emergency prepared for is not an emergency," and all possibilities had to be covered. For James Jackson Wiggins Brock, it was not enough to wear both belt and suspenders—I always suspected that he also pinned his trousers to his shirt.

After the sound of "3!" the room became completely silent for the briefest of moments, until the stentorian trumpeting of "ON!" and another cascade of arrhythmia proclaimed to the heavens and to us that the Brock finger was plunging into the valve. It stayed there only long enough for the chief to feel the nature of the obstruction and shout "OFF!", the declaration—along with the resumption of a normal heartbeat—of withdrawal back into the atrium. He announced that the leaflets were fused tightly together and the opening admitted only the very tip of his finger. A particularly forceful thrust would be required to free up the tissue and relieve the constriction. The need for such a maneuver certainly magnified the danger, but there was no other choice. Success would depend on Brock's ability to force the valve open without either causing an uncontrollable and therefore lethal irregularity of rhythm or cracking it so widely that retrograde flow up into the atrium would occur to cause worsening of the back pressure on the lungs. Such a serious regurgitation was even worse, if it is possible to imagine such a thing, than the stenosis itself. In other words, if Brock applied too little pressure, he would fail to sufficiently open the valve; if he applied just a bit too much, he would kill his patient.

Had Brock been a man who easily shared his anxieties for all to see, Fred would have no doubt leaned forward across the table at this point and *sotto voce* encouraged him with something like, "She's lucky you're her surgeon, Jim," or some similar proof of unquestioning confidence and solidarity. But saying something like that was tantamount to announcing to everyone in that room the unavoidable truth that was so obvious but must remain at all costs hidden—the chief's almost paralyzing fear of taking the next essential step in the operation. But the significant word here was *almost*. Whatever tremblings may have afflicted his courage as he paused there momentarily with his fingertip hovering above the straitened valve, none of us clustered around that operating table doubted that he would proceed. Though he could easily have declared the valve inoperable and retreated with a live but still critically ill patient, he would never do such a thing. As I would learn in later years, Brock was a man with an overpowering conscience, and his sense of responsibility would figuratively shout in his ear at moments like these. And of course, there across the table from him stood Fred, like a human gyroscope of stability. Not only that, but Fred's very presence was a challenge to action—and a demand, too.

The ultimate instant had now come. Not only was this my first meeting with a live human heart but it was also the first time I had ever been at an operation where a single maneuver might either cure or kill a patient, all within a period of a few seconds.

I was not optimistic. There were no effective anti-arrhythmic medications in 1954. Having just witnessed how badly this heart responded to the relatively minor stimulation of an exploring finger, I felt sure that any vigorous attempt to push the valve open would cause a problem so uncontrollable that death was certain. I was no longer spellbound by the heart's ineffable beauty. Though I continued to watch it carefully, my thoughts had again drifted off, this time out through the large swinging doors of the OR suite, to the small waiting room outside where Paul Stewart paced anxiously back and forth across the well-worn carpet.

I was yanked back by the stentorian sound of Dr. Brock trumpeting out the numbers as though their reverberation would reinforce his will: "1, 2, 3, ON!"—and he plunged his finger down into the valve orifice amid a staccato shower of violent irregularities in the heartbeat. It was like watching fireworks. The chief was standing on a stool now, and I could feel his upper arm against my shoulder. It moved slightly just then, and I sensed that he was about to withdraw his finger from the valve and back into the safety of the atrium, his job undone. The "OFF!" that now echoed through the room had a note of desperation in it. Brock looked across the operating table at his assistant and almost whined, as though he were on the verge of something near tears, "I can't do it, Fred. I just can't get my finger through the valve, dammit. It's too tight—I know I'll kill her if I keep pushing." And then plaintively, but in a way as though he was begging to be contradicted, "Now you wouldn't want me to try again and maybe kill her, would you, Fred?" and more insistently, "Would you?" But Fred would, and it was as though Brock had anticipated he would.

"Go ahead, Bill. I know you can do it. I've seen you crack tougher ones before. You have to try again." Fred spoke very gently, but his tone was firm. He was not to be denied. The words were precisely what Brock was asking for. As I watched it unfold over the few seconds it took, that scenario seemed not to be new. Perhaps it had been played out more than once before between the two men. The surgeon needed to be told that he must make another attempt. Without Fred, he might quit, and never forgive himself his failure. He had made the resident his appointed conscience, and all of us listening to their ex-change somehow knew it.

Fred had given his chief no choice, and no choice was just what Brock wanted. The chief mumbled something that was lost in his cloth mask, and I could feel his body steadying itself for the next move, as though in reflection of his stiffened resolve. Never having experi-enced such a situation before, I had no idea what to think. I knew only what lay behind Fred's urging: Better to lose this young woman's life in a vain attempt at cure than watch her die within the next few weeks by drowning in the backed-up fluid in her lungs. But I was far too in-experienced to understand the ineradicable feeling of guilt that goes with a death on the operating table. It would be years before I knew the intense loneliness of the surgeon when responsibility reaches such a magnitude; it would be years before I knew that the certainty of hav-ing no choice makes even the most wavering of captains become courageous.

Brock leaned into the table and I saw the top of his hand move as he began to advance his finger toward the bottom of the atrium and that unyielding valve. "1, 2, 3, ON!" He literally shouted it this time, while the heart started up its terrifying outburst of uncoordinated con-vulsions, as though little explosions were occurring all over the ventri-cles. As he hunched forward to press down into the valve, I suddenly felt something give, and the tightness in Brock's shoulder instantly re-laxed. The burst of release transmitted from inside the heart was so palpable that I believe I may not only have felt it but heard it, too. It was like a sudden pop, and though I had never before experienced it, I somehow knew that it was just right. There was something about the sensation of resistance overcome to tell me that Brock had expertly separated the leaflets without injuring their delicate structure. Instantaneously, the valve had become as close to normal as it was pos-sible to make it.

With "OFF!" the surgeon pulled his finger back into the atrium and the disordered rhythm stopped as suddenly as it had started. I felt as though I had experienced a miracle. I even began to imagine that the blood-choked lung was already becoming softer under my retractor. Perhaps I wasn't imagining it—it might well have been true.

Brock pulled his finger up out of the auricle, clamped the incision in its wall, and stepped down off the stool and away from the table, a broad grin wrinkling up his surgical mask. His blue eyes twinkled like a Santa Claus who had just delivered a particularly handsome and well-deserved gift. Though not very tall, standing there after that Olympian moment he seemed a giant. Fred looked over at him with genuine admiration, like a kid who has never really doubted that his older brother would beat up the schoolyard bully. Very quietly but obviously meaning it, he said—yes, he did say it—"She's lucky you're her surgeon, Jim."

It was the resident's turn to lower his finger into the valve, which he did with a respectful imitation of his chief's precautionary numbering. Having confirmed its near normalcy, he withdrew, sewed up the small opening in the wall of the auricle, and began to close the chest, as Dr. Brock went out toward the waiting room to give good news to Paul Stewart. Not a word was said about the moments of hesitancy.

When the dressing had been applied, our reviving patient was transferred back to her gurney and wheeled to the recovery room. By that time, she was wide awake and the breathing tube was ready to be removed. When it came out, I could scarcely believe the evidence before my eyes. This young woman, previously short of breath to the point of air hunger, was inhaling and exhaling as well as the nurse who stood by her bed. She lay almost flat on one pillow, and there was not a touch of blueness on her lips. The tears of despair had dried hours earlier, but when she became fully awake and realized that she had been given a new life, tears of joy appeared in their place. A fingertip had cured her, and also converted a third-year medical student into an acolyte of cardiac surgery.

I would, of course, go on to become Jim Brock's research fellow and then his resident, as had Fred before me. But somehow, it never felt completely comfortable. I finished all the training, was awarded a cardiac fellowship at the same renowned English hospital where the first European mitral valvulotomy had been done, and spent several years doing a series of heart cases as an attending surgeon, but my own heart was never wholly in it. From the beginning, I recognized that there was an intensity and single-mindedness in the psyche of cardiac surgeons that I did not share. I could not identify with them, could not see myself focused so totally on a single organ and a particular kind of surgical tour de force that excluded all others. And, of course, I had discovered the abdomen, a soft and welcoming place with a variety of vistas and challenges that suited the pace of my personality far better than did the high-risk, tightwire adventures that took place within the ribbed solidity of the chest's unyielding encasement. Abdominal surgeons are like me—they walk often among the commonest diseases, and thrive on jousting with their multiple complexities. They do seem to require great heights of attainment, but not as uninterruptedly as their cardiac colleagues—their need is not reawakened each day.

If the chest is a fortress that must be stormed in order to reach the rich pleasures within, then the abdomen has been for me a nurturing home of many variegated rooms, where my spirit may be tested, but is just as often nourished and expanded.

Still, I have never lost my fascination with the heart. Though it is no longer my household divinity, it has been like a first love, always in the background of my thoughts as she looked the very first time I saw her, but nowadays never the chief object of my devotion, or my desire.

CHAPTER EIGHT

THE HEART:

THE FIRST

AND LAST DYING

ASCINATION, such as I had at my first heart operation, may be the very word that best describes the basis for the idealized romance that not only I but men and women of every era have enjoyed with that most wondrous of organs. How far back does the enchantment go? Cave evidence exists of far more than the mere prehistoric awareness of the heart and its relationship to the blood—the earliest of our ancestors seem to have recognized that the very life force departs and the heart stops beating when large quantities of blood pour forth from the wounded body. On a wall of the cave of Pindal at Asturias in northern Spain may be seen the drawing of a mammoth, with a red heart that was ocherd into its center by a long-forgotten Paleolithic artist. Similar pictures have been found in the cavern of Niaux in southern France, of bisons with arrows imbedded in their chests at the location of the heart. Stone Age hunters must have known that this was the most direct way to kill an animal. Whether its victim was beast or man, the cave artists had doubtless witnessed the sight many times that Homer would sing of around 800

B.C.E., when he described the death of Alcathous at the hands of Idomeneus, in the *Iliad:* "And he fell with a thud, and the spear was fixed in his heart, that still beating made the butt thereof to quiver, till mighty Ares snuffed its fury out."

Not only in Paleolithic times but among many folk societies today, red indicates vigor and is therefore a much-favored color. Red ocher and other pigments have been found smeared on corpses discovered in French and Spanish burial caves, thought to have been applied before death in the hope of revivifying a failing man or woman. As recently as December 1998, archaeologists discovered the complete skeleton of a young child in a rock-shelter about 150 kilometers north of Lisbon. The child had been wrapped in a blanket or animal skin drenched in red ocher at some time prior to its ceremonial burial. Estimated to be twenty-eight thousand years old, the specimen indicates that even early humans apparently believed that blood incorporates the essence of life.

Since our species first developed the capacity to interpret the evidence of our senses and theorize about it, we seem to have perceived that life is associated with three overtly recognizable actions—movements, in fact—without which the body dies: breathing, the heartbeat, and the pulse. It is impossible to believe that man did not from his beginnings link them together in his conception of the differences between the quick and the dead, between the vital and the inert. To early man, there was no evidence of life without the three and without body heat. In the formulations of the early Greek physicians, the vital heat was said to originate in the heart. The heat, the heart, and the blood seem always to have been seen as inseparably associated.

More than 2500 years B.C.E., the physicians of Egypt had already developed a theoretical construct incorporating the importance of heartbeat, pulse, breathing, and body heat. With the discovery of certain papyri in the 1860s and 1870s (one in particular, the Ebers papyrus), historians have acquired some rather detailed knowledge of Egyptian beliefs about the body, going at least as far back as the period we now call the New Kingdom, from 1550 to 1070 B.C.E. Based on the well-documented conservatism of Egyptian thought, however, as well as certain clues in the text, it appears likely that most if not all of these formulations had existed with little change since the time of the Old Kingdom, 2649 to 2150 B.C.E.

The Egyptians believed the purpose of breathing to be the transport of air through the nostrils, down the windpipe, and then directly into the heart. Once having arrived there, the air and some water were said to be mixed into the blood, which passed from the heart into a series of ducts, called *metu,* for distribution to all parts of the body. Other *metu* flowing away from the organs and tissues were thought to carry their products or wastes—such as sweat, mucous, tears, semen, and urine—to appropriate locations on the body's surface, where they could be discharged. The Egyptians derived the notion of *metu* from their observation of certain cordlike structures of various lengths and diameters throughout the tissues. Though we now know that these were, in fact, arteries, veins, nerves, and tendons, neither the Egyptians nor other contemporaneous peoples distinguished among them.

The Egyptians considered the heart to be the most important organ of the body, not only while a person lived but after death as well. As in many civilizations of the time and before, it was their presumed site of origin of thought, emotion, and everything else that we moderns associate with the brain or mind. In fact, they had no word for mind—instead, they used "heart." For this reason, the heart was the site of conscience and one's character, and was destined to play an important role in the afterlife. Soon after the deceased enters the netherworld, according to this formulation, his heart, representing his conscience and character, is placed on a pan scale and measured against a feather, representing truth and order. Only if the heart weighs less than the feather is the deceased permitted to proceed in the afterlife. Because the heart was thus absolutely necessary to the welfare of the dead, it was the only organ left in place when a body was embalmed. All the others were stored in ceramic jars and buried with the corpse.

Proceeding outward from the heart as they did, the life-carrying *metu* were vital structures whose condition a doctor needed to know. He would evaluate them by feeling the pulse and in other ways attempting to examine tendons and those many strands situated close enough to the body's surface. The Ebers papyrus says of the heart:

> There are vessels from it to every part. As to this, when any physician . . . applies the hands or his fingers to the head, the back of the head, to the hands, to the location of the stomach, to the arms or to the feet, then he examines the heart, because all his parts possess its vessels.

Should any imbalance of air, water, or blood occur, the *metu* would transport the abnormality all through the body. Such imbalances were thought to be the cause of disease, much as similar problems would later be attributed by the Greeks to imbalances of the humors. So crucial to daily life was the condition of these presumed passageways that a common Egyptian greeting was "May your *metu* be sound."

There were also other ways by which disorders in the *metu* might cause illness. One of them was so prominent in Egyptian medical thinking that it bears special emphasis. When too much fecal matter accumulated in the lowermost part of the bowel, its putrefied contents—called *weheduw*—were said to enter the *metu* and contaminate the mixture of blood, water, and air. The dangerous fluid thus produced was able to force its retrograde way back to the heart, from where it would be distributed throughout the body, causing any of a variety of diseases.

Once in the *metu*, the *weheduw* took on the character of a puslike substance, which might then become visible in such locations as poorly healing wounds or bad teeth. In order to prevent the accumulation of *weheduw*, the average Egyptian indulged in the frequent use of cathartics, at least on three designated days each month. Enemas, too, were commonly employed for the same purpose, and are, in fact, believed to have been invented by the Egyptians during the First Dynasty.

Certain of the Egyptian physicians restricted their practices to specific parts of the body, such as eyes or teeth. Of these, one particularly important designation was Shepherd of the Anus, and it is not difficult to figure out why. In a system so focused on feces and its relationship to the heart, this particular specialist must have occupied a high position, at least professionally if not anatomically. In this usage, *anus* should no doubt be construed as "lower bowel," to include the final part of the colon and the rectum. This medical functionary's job was to do whatever was necessary in order to prevent the accumulation of *weheduw*. But there were limits beyond which even the Shepherd of the Anus could not stave off the inevitable. It was believed that absorption of poisonous material from the large bowel became impossible to combat as one became elderly. Dying of old age in Egypt meant having one's body destroyed by the *weheduw*.

Ridding oneself of the contaminating *weheduw* before it could work its way into the *metu* was the key to what we would now call preventive medicine. Because honey was thought to neutralize *weheduw* and prevent its reaching the heart, a common practice among the Egyptians was to stuff large quantities of the sweet, sticky stuff as high up into the rectum as it would go.

(Interestingly, it has long been known to modern physicians that honey has antibacterial properties: advantage is nowadays taken of this fact in the treatment of bedsores and other open contaminated wounds that are slow to heal. Very likely, the earliest Egyptian physicians had noted honey's salubrious effect on purulent open wounds and reasoned that it might be even more beneficial if applied directly at the rectal source. Or perhaps their use of it was due only to the association still invoked, of sweetness with goodness.)

Although honey packing was apparently unique to the Egyptians, "keeping the bowels open" is ageless advice, given to their charges by countless generations of physicians and grandmothers. Purging would take on a therapeutic life of its own with the Greek theory of humors, and in one form or another has never been erased from the list of home remedies recommended by healers of various sorts, from pagans to proctologists.

The fear of bowel stasis and poisoning by stool has been a recurrent theme throughout history. During the past century, it has been expressed in the form of a plethora of popular remedies, ranging from frequent enemas and high-colonic irrigations to a radical operation now thankfully fallen into disrepute, in which great lengths, or even all, of the colon were removed. The purpose of the fearsome surgery was to treat a fanciful syndrome called autointoxication, said to cause a variety of symptoms such as headache, backache, lassitude, poor appetite, and weight loss. In time, enthusiasts added certain diseases to the list of problems attributed to fecal self-poisoning, among them being tonsillitis, appendicitis, gallstones, diabetes, arthritis, tuberculosis, and some cancers.

This medical fad remained fashionable from its introduction in the 1890s until well into the 1930s, by which time it had become apparent that no evidence existed to support either the theory of autointoxication or the various therapies designed to combat it. It began to disappear from medical theory and practice, although it has, of course, remained with us in various forms to this day.

In addition to the urge to "take the waters," unsupported theories about the dangers of fecal intoxication, too, have been among the reasons for the centuries-long popularity of spas. In many of those vivifying venues, treatment went (and still goes) beyond watering the outside to watering the inside as well—beyond mineral baths to a cleansing procedure known euphemistically as internal lavage (alternatively called colon laundering), in which the lower bowel is washed out until the runoff is clear. With both internal and external surfaces thus purified, no disease dared come near. Symptoms were deterred, in a manner of speaking; no latter-day *weheduw* was permitted to force its way into the *metu* and back to the heart.

Although there is no definitive evidence that pre-Egyptian cultures concerned themselves with the dangers of accumulated stool, the widespread folk belief in the dangers of fecal autointoxication would seem to indicate that it is a near-universal phenomenon. The obsessive-compulsive streak in all of us appears to be imbedded in human nature. Contamination, purification, and salvation, whether physical or spiritual, are recurrent themes not only in magical thinking but in the great religions of the world as well. The kingdom of heaven is inherited only by those who approach with clean hands and a pure heart. In this sense, we are all Egyptians.

Physical degradation may be the wages of a constipated bowel, but moral degradation is the punishment for a constipated soul. Each, at least in the Egyptian scheme of things and in the scheme of many other early civilizations, came ultimately from the heart. Throughout history, the possessing of a pure heart has been celebrated as the salvation of the righteous:

> Who shall ascend into the hill of the Lord? or who shall stand in his holy place? He that hath clean hands, and a pure heart; who hath not lifted up his soul unto vanity, nor sworn deceitfully.

It seems always to have been understood—originally as fact, even if now only as metaphor—that moral, spiritual, emotional, and even sexual behavior and thoughts are attributable to the heart. The Hebrew word for heart, *lev*, appears 190 times in the Jewish Bible in a variety of connotations, summarized as though for a modern reader in a long paragraph to be found in the Talmudic tract *Midrash Rabbah*. In a commentary on Ecclesiastes 1:16, "I spoke with my own heart," the rabbinic authorities provide an extensive list of the moral, intellectual, and emotional involvements of the heart. In one long paragraph, they catalog virtually every property attributed, then or since, to the organ that William Harvey called "the source of all action":

> I SPOKE WITH MY OWN HEART (I, 16). The heart sees, as it is said, *My heart hath seen much.* It hears, as it is said, *Give Thy servant therefore a heart that hears* (I Kings III, 9). It speaks, as it is said, *I spoke with my own heart.* It walks, as it is said, *Went not my heart?* (II Kings V, 26). It fails, as it is said, *Let no man's heart fail within him* (I Samuel XVII, 32). It stands, as it is said, *Can thy heart stand?* (Ezekiel XXII, 14). It rejoices, as it is said, *Therefore my heart is glad and my glory rejoiceth* (Psalms XVI, 9). It cries, as it is said, *Their heart cried unto the Lord* (Lamentations II, 18). It is comforted, as it is said, *Bid Jerusalem take heart* (Isaiah XI, 2). It is troubled, as it is said, *Thy heart shall not be grieved* (Deuteronomy XV, 10). It becomes hard, as it is said, *The Lord hardened the heart of Pharaoh* (Exodus IX, 12). It grows faint, as it is said, *Let not your heart faint* (Deuteronomy XX, 3). It grieves, as it is said, *It grieved Him at His heart*

(Genesis XI, 6). It fears, as it is said, *For the fear of thy heart* (Deuteronomy XXVIII, 67). It can be broken, as it is said, *A broken and contrite heart* (Psalms LI, 19). It becomes proud, as it is said, *Thy heart be lifted up* (Deuteronomy VIII, 14). It rebels, as it is said, *This people hath a revolting and rebellious heart* (Jeremiah V, 23). It invents, as it is said, *Even in the month which he had devised of his own heart* (I Kings XII, 33). It cavils, as it is said, *Though I walk in the stubbornness of my heart* (Deuteronomy XXIX,18). It overflows, as it is said, *My heart overfloweth with a goodly matter* (Psalms XLV, 2). It devises, as it is said, *There are many devices in a man's heart* (Proverbs XIX, 21). It desires, as it is said, *Thou hast given him his heart's desire* (Psalms XXI, 3). It goes astray, as it is said, *Let not thy heart decline to her ways* (Proverbs VII, 25). It lusts, as it is said, *That ye go not about after your own heart* (Numbers XV, 39). It is refreshed, as it is said, *Stay ye your heart* (Genesis XVIII, 5). It can be stolen, as it is said, *And Jacob stole Laban's heart* (Genesis XXXI, 20). It is humbled, as it is said, *Then perchance their uncircumcised heart be humbled* (Leviticus XXVI,41). It is enticed, as it is said, *He spoke enticingly unto the damsel* (Genesis XXXIV, 3). It errs, as it is said, *My heart is bewildered* (Isaiah XXI, 4). It trembles, as it is said, *His heart trembled* (I Samuel IV, 13). It is awakened, as it is said, *I sleep, but my heart waketh* (Song of Songs V, 2). It loves, as it is said, *Thou shalt love the Lord thy God with all thy heart* (Deuteronomy VI, 5). It hates, as it is said, *Thou shalt not hate thy brother with thy heart* (Leviticus XIX, 17). It envies, as it is said, *Let not thy heart envy sinners* (Proverbs XXIII, 17). It is searched, as it is said, *I the Lord search the heart* (Jeremiah XVII, 10). It is rent, as it is said, *Rend your heart, and not your garments* (Joel II, 13). It meditates, as it is said, *The meditation of my heart shall be understanding* (Psalms XLIX, 4). It is like a fire, as it is said, *There is in my heart as it were a burning fire* (Jeremiah XX, 9). It is like a stone, as it is said, *I will take away the stony heart out of thy flesh* (Ezekiel XXXVI, 26). It turns in repentance, as it is said, *That turned to the Lord with all his heart* (II Kings XXIII, 25). It becomes hot, as it is said, *While his heart is hot* (Deuteronomy XIX, 6). It dies, as it is said, *His heart died within him* (I Samuel XXV, 37). It melts, as it is said, *The hearts of the people melted* (Joshua VII, 5). It takes in words, as it is said, *And these words, which I command thee this day, shall be upon thy heart* (Deuteronomy VI, 6). It is susceptible to fear, as it is said, *I will put My fear into their hearts* (Jeremiah XXXII, 40). It gives thanks, as it is said, *I will give thanks unto the Lord with my whole heart* (Psalms CXI, 1). It covets, as it is said, *Lust not after her beauty in thy heart* (Proverbs VI, 25). It becomes hard, as it is said, *He that hardeneth his heart shall fall into evil* (Proverbs XXVIII, 14). It makes merry, as it is said, *It came to pass when their hearts were merry* (Judges XVI, 25). It acts deceitfully, as it is said, *Deceit is in the heart of them that devise evil* (Proverbs XII, 20). It speaks from out of itself, as it is said, *Now, Hannah, she spoke in her heart* (I Samuel I, 13). It loves bribes, as it is said, *But thine eyes and thy heart are not but for covetousness* (Jeremiah XXII, 17). It writes words, as it is said, *Write them upon the table of thy heart* (Proverbs III, 3). It plans, as it is said, *A heart that deviseth wicked thoughts* (Proverbs VI, 18). It receives commandments, as it is said, *The wise heart will receive commandments* (Proverbs X, 8). It acts with pride, as it is said, *The pride of thy heart hath beguiled thee* (Obadiah 3). It makes arrangements, as it is said, *The preparations of the heart are man's* (Proverbs XVI, 1). It aggrandises itself, as it is said, *Will thy heart therefore lift thee up?* (II Chronicles XXV, 19). Hence, I SPOKE WITH MY OWN HEART, SAYING: LO, I HAVE GOTTEN GREAT WISDOM.

It is hardly necessary to add more. Still, perhaps a few everyday allusions common to our own time can serve to illustrate how persistently we cling to the metaphors in spite of our knowledge of modern physiology. In such ways is the richness of our language preserved and the ancient imagery of the heart not forgotten.

Even when the heart bleeds, it is not bleeding in the physical sense but in the metaphorical. Though many American presidents may have committed adultery, only one has confessed to doing it in his heart. Having made that admission, he ate his heart out over the unexpectedly negative—or perhaps heartless—public response, and felt heartsick and disheartened until the clamor died down. Some of us have hearts of gold, or of stone; warm or cold; we open our hearts to certain people, let them look into our hearts or join our hearts to theirs, but none of these seemingly surgical undertakings requires the use of an operating room to make it happen; the same is true for touching the heart, stirring it, breaking it or mending it; we continue to live though we have given our heart to another, or perhaps realize that it belongs to Daddy; the heart may be worn on the sleeve or leap unbidden into the mouth—it is a movable beast.

The heart and its vital redness have been intertwined with our conceptions not only of life but also of the origins of thought and emotion for as long as history provides records. It is not difficult to understand why a primitive mind should have assumed the connection. The heart can be felt to hasten, it skips, it even flutters; it is heavy, it is light, it sits at times like a lump in our throats or a weight in our chests; it seems literally to ache when we are sad and take wings when we are happy—no wonder that it was for tens of millennia thought to be the origin of emotions; no wonder that, even now when we know better, we continue to cling to the fable and cherish the romance of the heart's mythology.

Long before and long after the period when the Bible was being written, the Greeks followed in the tradition that the soul is associated with the heart. They listened almost three thousand years ago to the *Iliad,* as Homer described Sarpedon's death after the mighty Patroclus plunged a spear into his "solid heart."

> From the wide wound gushes out a stream of blood,
> And the soul issued in the purple flood.

The notion of the "solid heart," too, seems to have endured for millennia. Even the liver is not as firm as the muscle of the ventricles, and this firmness must have been interpreted as having great significance for the heart's role in human life. In the late sixteenth century, the French battlefield surgeon Ambroise Paré would describe what had long been accepted by those who had personal experience of that remarkable organ. He summed up in a single paragraph all of what was then believed by both physicians and the laity about the heart's role in the physical and spiritual life of mankind:

> The heart is the chief mansion of the Soule, the organe of the vitall
> faculty, the beginning of life, the fountain of the vitall spirits, and so

consequently the continuall nourisher of the vitall heat, the first living and last dying, which because it must have a naturall motion of itself, was made of a dense solide and more compact substance than any other part of the body.

The heart's solidity and the fact that it is cradled by a thin cushion of fluid within the fibrous envelope of pericardium were the reasons that the Hippocratic writings reflect certainty that the great organ is not subject to disease. The thesis that the heart is the beginning of life was certified by Aristotle, whose detailed studies of the developing chick embryo demonstrated unequivocally to him that the heartbeat is the first sign of life visible to the naked eye. Quite obviously, cardiac standstill was the ultimate evidence of death—the heart was "the first living and the last dying." That the heart is the source of the body's "vitall heat" was unquestioned by the Aristotelians, as it was unquestioned by every thinking person who accepted the basic tenets of Greek medicine.

But it was not enough for Aristotle that the heart should be merely the ruler of the body—he went further. In his system, based as it was on biology, the soul could not possibly be an entity completely independent of the body—it must arise from the heart, which he also considered to be the origin of the emotions and of intellect, although he did believe that this latter is mediated in some way through the brain. To Aristotle, his cardiocentric theory of life was unassailable: the heart beats of its own inner regulating mechanism; it is the obvious source of the innate heat; and it is even central in location. The evidence was overwhelming.

Plato and the school of Hippocrates, on the other hand, had located all intellectual faculties in the brain. By the end of the golden age of Greece, the battle had been joined that would be so clearly expressed more than a millennium and a half later in just two pithy lines of Shakespeare's *The Merchant of Venice,* uncharacteristically in four-legged meter:

> Tell me where is fancy bred,
> Or in the heart or in the head?

There are plenty of Shakespearean examples of fancy's origins in both, but a striking line is to be found in *The Tempest,* in which Prospero goes so far as to attribute one of the *heart's* physical characteristics to the *mind,* conflating the two in what would appear to be a unique way:

> a turn or two I'll walk,
> To still my beating mind.

The debate over heart versus head has never left us, although it has gradually come to be understood as a division of labor between the two, and in recent centuries a metaphoric one at that. Thus, we refer to the heart as our symbolic emotional center and the brain as the rational focus: "I listened to my heart instead of my head." These conceptions have been inherited from an intermediate mode of thinking in which the brain was acknowledged to be the site of intellectual functions but the heart maintained its authority over the emotions.

Sometimes the heart is replaced in metaphoric expressions by the stomach (the Egyptians, it will be recalled, referred to the stomach as "the mouth of the heart") or even the entire digestive tract, reflecting the old confusions about the two: "I don't have the stomach for it" or "I feel it in my gut." We even on occasion go so far as to assign the entrails an authority so dependable that it should overcome the mistaken dictates of the brain, as in "I have the gut sense that . . ."

As a result of the major scientific advances that were made in the seventeenth century—particularly William Harvey's discovery that the blood does not ebb and flow, as the Greeks would have it, but moves around the body in a circle driven by the pumping action of the heart—a considerable degree of rationality was invoked on theorizers who hoped to be taken seriously. As the real functions of various organs were being identified during the next 250 years, agreement became universal that the heart should be accorded no pretense of intellectual or emotional capacities.

But in a symbolic sense, the heart continued to maintain a kind of hegemony—especially in affairs of the heart. By this, I mean to imply not only romantic love but love for humankind as well. Perhaps of most significance, I refer to spiritual love. In the Christian tradition, the heart is both the province and provenance of divine love, and like all matters of faith, such a belief is independent of the need for bio-logic substantiation. The concept is metaphysical and not subject to the rules of scientific evidence. It is the heart of Christ—to some the Sacred Heart—and not his brain that is the centrality of divine love. Perhaps the very knowledge that thought and emotion really do arise in the brain paradoxically provides the symbolism with so much of its power. In this way of looking at it, the heart is the means of joining body and soul. Not only that, but as long as we continue—in spite of knowing that we do it metaphorically—to speak of emotions as though they come from the heart, we are using that organ to maintain a continuity between the present and the past.

Even in the face of science, the human mind has difficulty letting go of patterns of thought imprinted during civilization's earliest days. Sometimes, the reluctance is deliberate and enriching, as in the many metaphoric attributes of the heart. And sometimes the holding fast to ancient ways lies deep below the level of human consciousness. Like the neuroses that originate from early childhood perceptions, the transmitted effects of memory—shrouded as their origins may be— never leave our collective thinking; like individuals, cultures are made of memories, both the known and the hidden. Also as with individuals, departures from rational behavior are best understood by looking to the past for explanations and digging beneath the surface of everyday things.

Though they had no way of knowing that they were putting the cart before the horse (or the heart before the course), the ancients had physical evidence to support their certainty that emotions arose in the heart. We may interpret it differently, but that same evidence of such as fluttering or heavy hearts is available to us today. It provides an imagined justification for clinging to the comfortable tradition we ex-press so lyrically in our spoken words and in our literature. Emotions are, after all, not infrequently accompanied by sensations in the front of the chest, often arising in the heart itself. Like early man, we too are aware of skipped beats, changes in rate, and vague sensations of cardiac distress, including those that arise from stress-related reflux of stomach acid into the lower esophagus, or a spasm of that tubular structure. We may knowingly mistake the effect for the cause, but heartache is sometimes real. Every person who has ever suffered from any degree of depression has felt the weight in his chest, and knows the meaning of "My heart is heavy."

So our expressions are based on more than imagination. It has long been recognized that pulse rate and blood pressure can change with changing mood. And recent studies of the physiological effects of emotions indicate that there are often distinct cardiac responses to such feelings as anger and depression. Not only rhythm but even the pattern of contraction of the ventricles and their output of blood appear to depend somewhat on state of mind, as does the secretion of certain hormones and neurotransmitters. Although much research remains to be done—and less attention has been paid to happier feelings—it may very well be that such expressions as "heavy-hearted," "light-hearted," and even "chicken-hearted" have a basis in real events going on in the cardiac muscle and chambers, events that the conscious mind can sense. Like us, the ancients had their reasons.

So much, at least for the moment, for the origins of present-day cardiac metaphor and symbolism. What about structure and function; what about the development of knowledge of the heart that we think of as scientific, and therefore rational? For this, it is necessary to turn to the glory days of Alexandria, where a great medical school was founded in approximately 300 B.C.E., only a short time after Alexander and Aristotle died within a year of each other, in 323 and 322 B.C.E. respectively.

Following the death of Alexander, Egypt fell under the control of one of his generals, Ptolemy, who established a dynasty that would last until the death of Cleopatra in 30 B.C.E. Like every central city of a great empire, Alexandria became the cosmopolitan beneficiary of intellectual and commercial enterprise and was the hub of Hellenic culture. It was in that thriving and tumultuous place that systematic dissection of the human body was carried out for the first time. So in-

tent were the physicians of the Alexandrian school on learning the secrets of anatomy and physiology that they very likely even went so far
as to vivisect condemned criminals, although this probability has
never been substantiated by incontrovertible evidence.

By discovering the cardiac valves and also demonstrating that there
is a distinction between the thick-walled arteries and the thin-walled
veins, the physicians of Alexandria made two enormous contributions
to the understanding of the heart. In keeping with the theories of the
time involving pneuma and nutrition, they believed that it is the function of veins to carry nourishing blood out from the liver, while the arteries transport the vital spirit from the heart. Spirit, or pneuma,* had
long been thought to be brought in from outside by the act of breathing, and then transformed into one or another variant of itself. In contrast to Aristotle, who taught that the body has within it an innate
pneuma, the Alexandrians taught that the pneuma, having been
drawn into the lungs during inspiration, was passed on to the heart,
where it became vital spirit. The vital spirit was then said to be propelled out to the body via the arteries. Not only did this mean that the
lungs, heart, and arteries formed a single continuous respiratory system, but also that the arteries contained only spirit and no blood. The
spirit that reached the brain was said to be converted there into another form of itself, called psychic spirit.

The Alexandrians were the first to recognize the significance of the
nervous system as the center of the body's organization. So sophisticated was their understanding that they distinguished between nerves
that carry sensation (now called sensory nerves) and those that carry

---

To avoid confusion, I treat the words pneuma *and* spirit *as though they are interchangeable here, recognizing that there were sometimes subtle—and very occasionally significant—differences in certain usages. In Chapter 5, I discussed the equally subtle differences
between the concepts of soul, psyche, and anima. All three are dependent on the notion of
pneuma or spirit somehow entering the body from outside, and ultimately from the cosmos. One
should not rack one's brain with these abstruse and often indistinct interrelationships. The
Greeks were often just as unclear about them as any modern reader has a right to be.*

messages activating muscles (now called motor nerves). In their conception, it was the psychic spirit acting through those nerves that made things happen. The central nervous system was thus seen as the organizing mechanism of the body, while the arteries brought vital spirit and the veins provided nourishment.

Since the arteries contained only vital spirit, it was necessary to explain why they bled when cut. To solve this dilemma, the Alexandrian physicians dreamed up a series of nonexistent connections between the arteries and the veins, through which blood was said to be transferred as soon as injury occurred. This imaginative thesis of imaginary connections went unquestioned for almost five hundred years, until Galen came along and disproved it by a simple experiment, which he repeated many times in public. He would place two ties a short distance apart around the circumference of an artery in a living animal, thereby isolating the segment of vessel. He would then isolate the artery from other structures to show that it had no connections to nearby veins. Then he would cut across it, releasing the blood that he had thereby shown to have been present before the incision was made.

The Alexandrian emphasis on direct study of human anatomy was destined not to last. The influence of their example seems to have disappeared when the physicians of the school were expelled by the Ptolemy who ruled during the latter half of the second century B.C.E. There is no record of systematic human dissection from then until it was again taken up in Italy during the late fifteenth century. In fact, medical progress in general bogged down after the Alexandrian period, with the single exception of Galen, who was born in Asia Minor in 129 C.E. By the time of his death in 201, Galen had established himself—through a combination of talent and self-promotion—as the ultimate authority on all things medical.

Until the middle of the sixteenth century—and to a gradually diminishing degree for almost three hundred years afterward—Galen's teachings on anatomy reigned supreme, even though they were based on the dissection of small animals, among which his favorite was the macaque monkey. His hoary hold did not weaken until the publication of Vesalius's great book in 1543, which demolished several of the old doctrines at a single blow and began the long and circuitous journey toward truly scientific study.

Galen's ideas of the body were a combination of time-honored theories (particularly those of the Hippocratic school) and the observations he made during the dissection and vivisection of his animals. His physiology was thus a strange mix of fact and fancy made all the more confusing to a modern reader by his tendency to sometimes misinterpret the evidence of his own eyes in order to fit it into a predetermined pattern. On other occasions, though, his interpretations were direct and accurate. One example of this is the way in which he approached the old belief that because speech seems to come from the chest, its source must be the heart. Since one cannot speak without thinking, the ancients reasoned that thought must originate in the heart rather than the brain. The cardiocentric Aristotle, of course, believed this. To dispute it, Galen cut the nerves to the vocal cords of a live pig (these are the recurrent laryngeal nerves, which can be traced directly to their source in the vagus nerve that originates in the base of the brain). The pig's squeals were immediately hushed to a bare whisper, which he interpreted as proving that the brain, and not the heart, is the origin of the voice and therefore of thought.

As noted earlier, Galen was convinced of the earlier idea that the liver, being the structure that makes the blood, is also the site from which it is distributed to the tissues of the body. By the ebb and flow thesis to which he subscribed, each organ takes what it requires as the blood reaches it via the veins, after which the residue recedes with the tide. This meant that a large quantity of blood constantly had to be replenished by the liver in order to replace the considerable used-up portion.

Galen dealt with the heart and lungs in a truly innovative way. Noting that the tissue of the lung was light and delicate, he decided that ordinary liver-made blood reaching it by passing unchanged through the right side of the heart was too heavy for its nourishment. He therefore decided that the blood must undergo a second coction on its way through the heart, to make it sufficiently light for the frothy substance of the lung.

Having invented this novel scheme, Galen was left with the riddle of explaining the ancient necessity that the body be vivified by the spirit, pneuma, or soul taken in from the outside with each respiration. Moreover, he had to get the spirit into the arteries that he had shown to contain blood. Since the arteries were part of the Greek concept of the respiratory system and were not connected with the liver, he had to dream up a way to explain how both spirit and blood got into them. Never at a loss, resourceful Galen made up a scheme. He agreed with contemporary doctrine that the inspired air passed from the lung into the left ventricle. Here it was transformed into vital spirit, warmed by the innate heat, and passed out into the arteries, which therefore contained life itself. But to explain the presence of blood—that was the difficulty in this confabulated formulation.

Galen had to figure out some way to get blood into the left ventricle to mix with the vital spirit being made there from the inspired air. This was a particularly challenging problem, since he and his predecessors conceived of the respiratory system of spirit and the nutritive system of blood as being independent of each other. Being the inventive fellow he was, he asserted that there were minute pores in the wall, or septum, separating the two sides of the heart, in order to allow blood to pass into the left ventricle. In fact, he claimed to have seen them.

The Galenic theory of circulation, then, may be summarized as follows: All blood is manufactured in the liver. Most of it goes out via the veins to nourish the body, by means of an ebb and flow motion. Other veins carry a smaller amount of blood up into the right ventricle, to be lightened before proceeding to the lungs. A fraction of it passes directly into the left ventricle through the imaginary pores that Galen invented because he had to figure out a way in which the two chambers might be shown to communicate with each other. From there, the mixture of vital spirit and blood goes out to the body through the arteries.

Galen's inventiveness did not stop there. Because he believed in the Alexandrian concept that *psychic* spirit is produced in the brain, he had to explain how this spirit was manufactured from the *vital* spirit that reached that organ via the arteries from the heart. Even this formidable task did not faze him. He postulated that on reaching the base of the skull, the vital spirit entered a network of blood vessels he claimed to have found there, which he called the *rete mirabile*. The transformation, he asserted, begins in the *rete mirabile* and is completed in the brain. From there, the psychic spirit is passed out through the nerves, which can accept it because they are hollow.

The entire formulation was bought—*in toto*—by the physicians of the time, and transmitted by them to many generations of their successors. It would be almost fifteen hundred years before Vesalius showed that, like other critical aspects of Galen's anatomy and physiology, neither the *rete mirabile* nor the pores were verifiable. They simply did not exist. The accurate observations of Vesalius, plus the discovery that veins contain valves that permit flow in only one direction, enabled William Harvey to begin the process of thought that would lead in the third decade of the seventeenth century to the discovery that, as he so succinctly summarized it:

> It must therefore be concluded that the blood in the animal body moves around in a circle continuously, and that the action or function of the heart is to accomplish this by pumping.

Harvey's proof was straightforward and understandable by any literate person who would take the time to think about it. He measured the output of each heartbeat, calculated the volume of blood leaving the heart per unit of time, and pointed out that it was impossible for a day's worth to be manufactured by the liver. Since the direction of flow was centrifugal in the arteries and centripetal in the veins (as shown by the configuration of the valves), the only explanation that was consistent with all observations was that blood moves in a circle, propelled only by the pumping of the heart.

Like Galen, Harvey was left with some gaps that needed to be filled, quite literally in fact. He was at first unable to explain how, in order to return to the heart, blood passes from the smallest peripheral arteries of the tissues and organs into the smallest veins. But *un*like Galen, he solved his problem not with a leap of imagination but a leap of confidence—confidence, that is, in the accuracy of his own observations and the detached way in which he had interpreted them. As Claude Bernard would teach two centuries later, he based his scientific imagination on evidence he had derived scientifically. The evidence of his experiments having convinced him that there simply had to be some sort of connecting channels carrying blood between the terminal portions of the arteries and the beginning of the veins, he predicted that they would one day be found. Eschewing the example of his boastful predecessor in yet another way, he made no claim to have seen them. In 1660, Marcello Malpighi of Bologna would justify his certainty by discovering the capillaries.

But in spite of Harvey's great discovery, the role of inspired air—the fabled pneuma—remained obscure. It had long been observed that blood leaving the exposed lung of an experimental animal is redder than blood entering it, but no one was quite sure why. Until Harvey's studies, the function of breathing was still thought to be twofold: it introduced pneuma or air to generate the vital spirit and it cooled the blood emanating from the source of innate heat, the heart. It was our melancholic friend Richard Lower who brought clarity to the problem by direct experiments on the source of the reddening phenomenon in 1669. Injecting venous blood directly into the vessels entering a living animal's lung, he observed that the dark fluid turned bright red as the lung took in air. He correctly assumed that the change occurred because of "the penetration of particles of air into the blood." He hypothesized that the blood became darker as the "particles of air" were lost from it during its subsequent passage through the tissues. It would later be shown that the critical constituent of the air is oxygen, a gas that was isolated only three years after Lower made his own Harvey-like leap of confidence.

Harvey's and Lower's conjectures were based on objectively interpreted experiment without the construction of a preconceived grand scheme of human biology into which they were forced to fit. Galen's, on the other hand, was conjecture based on fantasy, dreamed up to fill empty spaces in an edifice that was intended to hold an uneasy mix of real observation and baseless theory, built according to some imagined all-comprehensive plan designed by a divine architect. Harvey's contribution began with small and meticulous observations that ineluctably led to a hypothesis. His analysis was constructed entirely of verifiable observations whose interpretation he never distorted to squeeze into a preordained shape. When his theory emerged lacking only a single substantiating observation, he knew where that observation would be found, since his case had been so strongly built that it was, in a manner of speaking, watertight. His work represented not only a triumph of inductive reasoning but a highly visible departure from the human predisposition to invent explanations for the experienced phenomena of nature. Whether the inventing had a mystical basis as it did for the early folk societies who saw sprites and spirits in every wind and tree, or had a religious underpinning as it did for van Helmont, or was part of a campaign of self-promotion and personal theology as in the case of Galen, the result was nevertheless spurious and without evidence to support it.

With William Harvey began the modern understanding of the heart. He was the quintessential researcher of his age, the first truly glorious century in the history of science and in the critical analysis of nature. Not until that time did observers of natural phenomena overcome their need to produce huge overarching "theories of everything." From then on, the old habits would be increasingly replaced by the recognition that only by making small observations of small phenomena would the great patterns of nature ever emerge and be fully disclosed. Though René Descartes never wholly freed himself from unfounded speculation, he did express the mood of the new era when he wrote, "But like a man walking alone in the darkness, I resolved to proceed so slowly and carefully that, even if I did not get very far, I was certain not to fall." The old tendency to attempt progress by making great airborne leaps directly to the finish line was now giving way to the realization that small and steady steps were more accurate and certain.

By following Harvey's example of the keen observation of small things; by dispassion; by the search for bits of quantitative evidence; by critical analysis and interpretation; and by inductive reasoning, the process of discovery was soon under way whereby not only the structure and function of the heart would be elucidated, but that of every other organ and tissue of the body. Laboratory researchers concern themselves far less these days with organs and tissues than with cells and intracellular phenomena, but the method of science has remained the same. It can be summed up in a single sentence written by Harvey in 1653:

> Nature herself must be our advisor; the path she chalks must be our walk. For as long as we confer with our own eyes, and make our ascent from lesser things to higher, we shall be at length received into her closet-secrets.

The study of the heart had become scientific in the seventeenth century. Not only was the organ's normal function being elucidated, but its diseases were coming to be better understood. At the same time, the study of disease in general was beginning to be approached in new ways, based on correlating symptoms with the underlying pathological changes causing them, as discovered at autopsy. In 1761, a seventy-nine-year-old Italian anatomist, Giovanni Morgagni, published a massive study in five volumes, doing just that in a total of seven hundred patients whose bodies had been examined after death. The publication of that book, called in English *The Seats and Causes of Disease,* stimulated a great surge of interest in medical diagnosis, as physicians armed with the new knowledge found ever better ways to determine the diseased condition of internal organs by physical examination and the narrative of illness. The aim of diagnosis became to use the symptoms as related by the patient and the findings of physical examination to determine the nature of the pathological changes that had occurred within the body.

The invention of the stethoscope in 1816 allowed a great step forward in these endeavors. The heart and lungs became the object of medical scrutiny as never before. Curiosity about the basis of cardiac activity generated research by committed physicians during the nineteenth century trying to determine whether the heartbeat is initiated by stimuli from nerves or by some mechanism inherent within the organ itself. Ever since Galen had shown that the excised heart of an animal continues to beat on its own, the so-called myogenic (generated in the muscle) theory had been debated. "The power of pulsation has its origin in the heart itself . . . It does not need the nerves to perform its function," Galen had written in one of his more objective and realistic moments, but later authors did not necessarily agree, especially after medical thought had been freed from his stranglehold. As medicine became ever more scientific during the late eighteenth and early nineteenth centuries, voices were raised in favor of a neurogenic theory, a theory, that is, based on the conduction of impulses entering the heart via the nerves.

The controversy continued until a series of experiments conducted by English investigators between the 1860s and 1890s provided definitive evidence for a myogenic theory. Finally in 1907, Arthur Keith and Martin Flack of London described their discovery of the sinoatrial, or SA, node, a tiny collection of specialized muscle cells situated in the back wall at the top of the right atrium, which serves as a pacemaker to generate and drive the coordinated beat of the heart. Originating in the SA node, messages are carried by an arborizing bundle of other specialized muscle cells forming fibers to a relay station between the atrium and the ventricles, called the atrioventricular, or AV, node. From there, the electrical impulse is transmitted downward to the wall of the ventricles, causing them to contract. It is this electrical activity that is recorded when an electrocardiogram is done. No nerves are required to initiate it. In this case, Galen was right.

In fact, electrocardiography can trace, as it were, its beginnings to this period of time as well. In 1903, Willem Einthoven, a professor of physiology at the University of Leiden, published the results of experiments in which he had adapted a string galvanometer to record the currents generated by the heart. Over the next quarter century, he continued to add contributions that established the field of electrocardiography, and eventually brought Joe Boylan and me face to dumbstruck face with Jake the Janitor.

The latter half of the twentieth century has witnessed previously unimaginable advances in cardiology, both for diagnostic and therapeutic methods. Even a procedure as seemingly chimerical as cardiac transplantation has been routinely performed for some fifteen years. At this writing, researchers are beginning to report that they may one day stimulate embryonic stem cells to specialize into heart muscle in order to renew tissue damaged by disease. There seems no end to the possibilities inherent in the benisons promised by the science of cardiology.

Almost 375 years have passed since William Harvey launched the new way of thinking about the heart. The unfounded speculations and imaginary pores and spirits invoked by his lengthy line of predecessors have been discarded, as have the thought patterns that led to their promulgation. We have long known that the heart is not the seat of the emotions, and we think of the spirit in ways that the old Greeks would not recognize. And yet we remember, not only in our conscious minds but buried deeply within some subterranean chamber from which it sometimes finds its way to awareness, that the belief in magical forces once lived and will always live within us. Though our rational selves no longer believe in them, we find comfort sometimes in returning to the childhood of civilization and invoking, even if only in our language and legend, symbolism from the past.

But the symbolism of the past intrudes itself still into our perceptions. Magical thinking, the tendency to invent nonexistent structures and energies in order to create a reality that has never existed, the need to believe that wishing or fearing will make it so—these are matters we must be aware of. They are inherent predispositions—perhaps they might even be called instincts, or at least drives—that will ever be with us. It is because they are so deeply woven into human nature that we often feel more comfortable with them than we do with the harsh and relatively modern light of rationality.

The old ways are friends of imagination. Used well, they can be friends of creativity, too, so long as we recognize them for what they are, and travel only short distances with them. We must never allow ourselves to forget that metaphor and symbol serve us best when we bear in mind that they are only proxies for truth.

CHAPTER NINE

THE UTERUS:

THE HYSTERICAL

PASSION

No matter the confusion of mystical, speculative, and real that characterized early notions about the viscera, there is at least a certain consistency in the way each organ's activities were understood—or misunderstood—in any era and place. As civilizations became more coherent and structured, so did their theories of the body and its parts. Though it would be a mistake to assume that any firm unity was achieved among the various beliefs held by the many different peoples of many different periods, all of them did share two similar features: each reflected the characteristics of its own distinctive milieu; and there was considerable cross-pollination of concepts over a broad spectrum of societies and times.

With the advent of the Hippocratic era about four centuries B.C.E., a new ingredient entered the mix: remarkably accurate and systematic observations of the body's behavior in health and disease, divorced from explanations dependent on supernatural influence. The Greeks *saw* blood, phlegm, and yellow bile; they *convinced themselves* that black bile exists. To them, these were concepts that were free of supernaturalism as opposed to the Aesculapian system they replaced, in which the gods caused disease and patients went to a temple to be cured. From that period onward, and until the time of Galen, informed people—at least those affected by Greek culture—acquired their notions of what goes on inside themselves by accepting various elements of the uneasy confederation of three components. The trio consisted of the formalized conceptions of the Hippocratics and other groups of trained doctors; the heritage of earlier philosophers (of whom Empedocles was the most prominent), offering overarching theories of the macrocosm and microcosm; and the persistent magical beliefs of earlier peoples and the common folk. The three elements comprised a generalized body of thought, some of it valid and much of it fanciful, but nevertheless in harmony with the belief systems of a wide spectrum of Hellenic society, each part of the troika affecting the other two in intangible but definite ways.

Late in the second century C.E., Galen would from this triple stream of sources codify his own system of anatomy and physiology, which would become a powerful influence over the thinking of physicians and other more or less educated people for almost a millennium and a half. Although his formulations were based less on the verifiable truths he was able to add to the sum of medical theory than on the tried and untrue values of philosophy and imagination, his painstaking observations and experiments nevertheless made it possible to come closer than before to a general comprehension of the body's internal workings. Had they been properly followed up in the next centuries, his contributions and even his errors might have served as a basis upon which further clarifications could be constructed and new knowledge acquired.

But it was not to be. The magisterial Galen's uncontested authority and the intellectual sluggishness of the medieval period essentially shut down further creative medical thought until the late fifteenth century. During all the intervening time, the overbearing force of Galen's enormous oeuvre (amounting to the equivalent of some twenty-two thick octavo volumes of closely printed material) maintained the domination of a medicine based on two principles, both of which were considered beyond questioning. The first was the thesis that health and even basic constitution are determined by the balance of the four humors. The other is the certainty that divine purpose not only guides the functions of the organs but determines the details of their structure as well. Though the Hippocratics had been meticulous about excluding religious or magical influences from their reckoning of health, the enduring power of Galen's teachings would, half a millennium later, reestablish the primacy of a guiding afflatus, although there might be disagreements about His or its nature. The new religion of Christianity was very much at ease with such a concept, as was the old religion of the Jews. The theory of humors and the reliance on spiritual and other nonverifiable energies to explain biological phenomena would continue to be a factor in medical thought until almost two hundred years ago.

The belief in undemonstrated forces died a slow and sputtering death. It lived on well beyond its time, most ironically in the conceptions of some of those whom we and their contemporaries have held up as personifications of the objective scientist. Even that master of experimentalism William Harvey did not hesitate to express his belief that the heartbeat is initiated by some kind of unclassifiable energy inherent in the forcefulness of the blood entering the atrium. Whether in the form of such immeasurable forces or spiritual powers of celestial origin, the adherence to nonmaterial vitalistic explanations pervaded biological thinking until well into the nineteenth century.

But in looking back on all of this, one comes away with at least some sense of order. Following upon Galen's formulations, there was even a kind of logic to it. If the two basic premises—divine handiwork and the influence of the humors—were embraced, almost all of what flowed from them seemed acceptable to a rational mind. And that was one of the distinctions that Church leaders were attempting to make between their own teachings and the practices of superstition—between systems of thought that are acceptable to a mind accustomed to rational deliberation and those that appeal to one that allows itself to run with the sprites and elves. Though the fathers of the early and medieval Church were themselves saturated with residual superstition, they did what they could to make the distinction. In their renowned fifteenth-century statement concerning sorcery, devil worship, and the like, *Malleus maleficarum,* the two Dominican witch-hunters Heinrich Kramer and James Sprenger quoted a scriptural gloss in which appears the defining assertion that "Superstition is undisciplined religion, that is, religion observed with defective methods in evil circumstances." Although theologians of today would go far further in separating the divine from the magical, the underlying message is nevertheless the same—once having been stripped of any lingering absurdities, true religious belief should be the product of minds accustomed to reason.

Religion involves a faith that is systematized. If one conforms to certain basic principles, all consequent belief flows logically from them. This was what the fathers of the early Church were attempting to promulgate. They were convinced that they had separated themselves from magic and paganism, closing their eyes to all the residuum of earlier practices with which their own rituals and dogmas were permeated. Parallels can obviously be drawn between the tenets of Christianity and the systematized theoretics of Galenism. Both creeds purported to have thrown off the yoke of superstition and replaced it with the stability of revealed truth. The ideal nutritive ambience for Galenic thought was an atmosphere in which the hegemony of the Church was continually growing.

Both Galenism and the Church relied on the conviction that a scripture, a theology, the enduring influence of powerful founders, and the guidance of a single deity protected them from making the errors of those they considered primitives. In this conviction, they were often wrong. Plenty of instances of this kind of error are to be found in the early and medieval church as well as the annals of medical theory, even well beyond the period of Galenic hegemony. Some of them will be apparent in the remainder of these pages, as they have already been throughout this narrative.

But notwithstanding the consistency and structure of medical scripture and theology that existed even in ancient times, there was one biological area into which little or no logic or system seems to have intruded. To the bewildered perceptions of early man (and sometimes even to the sophisticated modern), what could be more unknown, unexplainable, and even on occasion terrifying than the visible, palpable sex organs? What a show they put on! They appear to have minds of their own, lusts of their own, even moment-to-moment physical changes of their own, over which no man or woman has predictable control. The genitals of both sexes tingle and become engorged; they fill with hot pulsing blood or lie flaccid and drained; they rise up of their own volition or recede when they no longer care; they spurt or ooze wetnesses or they remain dry; they draw us into each other's arms or make us turn away repelled; they lure us with seductive promise of joyful fulfillment, and even compel actions we would not otherwise consider; they serve up sensations sublime that demand contortions ridiculous; they elevate us to the highest of spiritual planes and sometimes bring us crashing down to the lowest of degradations; they enable victories unobtainable without their complicity, and the urgency of their importunate demands has brought disaster to individuals and nations— all without allowing us the freedom of choice that characterizes all of our other conscious actions. Certainly, the sex organs are different.

No wonder that long after humans abandoned much of their baseless conjecture about animals within and similar attempts to explain other aspects of nature, they continued to cling to magical theories about the genital structures, and in time came to justify some of their flights of fancy by calling them science. And no wonder that plenty of evidence exists of every generation's thralldom to the power of genital symbolism. Statuettes as ancient as the Old Stone Age have been unearthed that demonstrate great artifice of form and enhancement in order to emphasize penises, vulvas, and secondary sexual characteristics, such as breasts and buttocks. And no wonder, too, that the labia and phallus figure so prominently among the magical and healing artifacts of so many cultures. Even today, for example, when strolling the downtown streets of my home city on a summer's evening I will not infrequently encounter at least one or two men who appear to be of southern Italian extraction, wearing phallic amulets around their necks to let the world know of their virility. Though the dangling objects are said to be in the configuration of a water buffalo's horn (in it-self highly suggestive), there can be no doubt about their origin. The prevalence of necklaces strung with labia-shaped seashells is a re-minder that such objects were used for similar purposes long, long ago. The genitals have that of the mystical about them.

Symbolic representations of the magical qualities of the visible sex-ual apparatus will almost certainly remain overtly or subtly interwoven with cultural patterns as long as our species exists. There seems never to have been a time when the external organs of sex were not thought to act on their own, determining behavior and causing consequences that change lives—affecting the way we think and the emotions left be-hind long after they have ceased to work their turbulent willfulness on us. Our unremembered forebears saw them as capricious creatures in and on their bodies, but not wholly *of* them. They attributed all man-ner of magic to them, and pondered the lore of penises and vulvas un-governable or in servitude to demonic powers that instruct their erratic flights, whether of determined purpose or mere whimsy.

If such ruminations were evoked by the reproductive parts that can be seen, what must have been thought of those invisible—and there-fore even more mysterious? The unbridled heat of passion yields in the general course of events to the tranquil fruitfulness of the womb; the frenzy of sexual climax leads to the harmonious fecundity of the structure known to the Greeks as *hystera* and to the Romans as *matrix* (from *mater,* for mother and "motherhood"). The temptress is trans-formed into the mother, the seductress becomes the madonna. But the lack of control remains. Even the logic-besotted Greeks believed the generative organs to be at times beyond the power of the divine psyche to influence. Plato said of them that they are "disobedient and self-willed," demanding always to perform their lascivious function re-gardless of contrary instructions from the higher parts of the body. The entire schizophrenic calculus of sexuality and its outcomes was beyond the understanding of the men and women of earliest times. It remains incompletely solved even today. There are those romantics, I among them, who believe that this may not be such a bad thing.

Given that the role—and even the existence—of the ovary was for

so long not known, the most concealed organ of sexuality and reproduction was the uterus, as the Romans called the womb (from *uter,*
meaning "a bag"). Whether as *hystera, matrix,* or what we call it today,
the uterus continued to mystify mankind for millennia. One of the
reasons for the mystification was simply the traditional notion that secret visceral goings-on were constantly occurring deep within the re-
cesses of the abdomen, involving all inner structures. Unexplained
rumblings and gurgles could be felt and heard from down there, and
there were the occasional high-pitched squeals. And there was certainly movement. Were the viscera communicating in some way,
whether with one another or with something in the outside world?
Was there an unknowable argot, which if only understood might con-
vey messages that were not meant to be intercepted by men?

But of all the internal organs, the uterus was the one whose activities seemed most fraught with obscure significance. Its sexual and reproductive associations made it a thing of witchcraft and internal
animism. It was said to roam the inside of women's bodies, now with
slow deliberation, now leaping from place to place. It went where it
wanted and did what it wanted; it had secrets of its own and moods of
its own. When it wished, it could be a troublemaker. Some, such as
Plato, it will be remembered, called it an animal within an animal.

In *Timaeus* the great philosopher said of the uterus that it resembles
an animal intent on bearing children. "When it remains unfertilized
for a long time during the proper season the uterus becomes seriously
angry and moves all over the body; by obstructing the outlets of the
pneuma it prevents respiration, throws the patient in confusion and
provokes a variety of other diseases."

The Hippocratic physicians inherited these notions from centuries
of their predecessors, who in turn learned them from earlier tribal beliefs. In disavowing mysticism, the Hippocratics rejected any idea of
spiritual forces activating the uterus, but they could not completely
free themselves from the certainty that—although they denied magical incitement—the *hystera* did nevertheless move a bit, at least within
the confines of the pelvis. Many of their medical contemporaries went
further. They were convinced that the organ was able to pass through

the diaphragm and travel as high as the throat. When dehydrated, it was said to fling itself at the liver in order to be moistened by humors. When overheated, it leaped toward the coolness of the outside air. For centuries before and after those days of Hippocrates, the consequences of its peregrinations were thought to be dire.

Witness the following second-century C.E. statement by one of the most prominent physicians of his time, Aretaeus the Cappadocian, whose methods and teachings were closer to Hippocratic principles than were those of any of his contemporaries, not excluding Galen himself. In spite of this, he was nevertheless certain of the unpredictability of uterine wandering. Almost an entire pertinent chapter is here quoted from his extant works, in order that the full flavor may be tasted of what was during his time generally accepted as the behavior of the uterus. And this by an observer who rejected any thought of supernatural influence on the body. Aretaeus entitled this chapter "On Hysterical Suffocation."

> In the middle of the flanks of women lies the womb, a female viscus, closely resembling an animal; for it is moved of itself hither and thither in the flanks, also upwards in a direct line to below the cartilage of the thorax, and also obliquely to the right or to the left, either to the liver or spleen; and it likewise is subject to prolapsus downwards, and, in a word, it is altogether erratic. It delights, also, in fragrant smells, and advances toward them; and it has an aversion to fetid smells, and flees from them; and, on the whole, the womb is like an animal within an animal.
>
> When, therefore, it is suddenly carried upwards, and remains above for a considerable time, and violently compresses the intestines, the woman experiences a choking, after the form of epilepsy, but without convulsions. For the liver, diaphragm, lungs and heart, are quickly squeezed within a narrow space; and therefore loss of breathing and of speech seems to be present. And, moreover, the carotids [the carotids are the major arteries to the brain, running from the chest up to the base of the skull] are compressed from sympathy with the heart, and hence there is a heaviness of head, loss of sensibility, and deep sleep. . . .

If, therefore, upon the womb's being moved upwards, she begins to suffer, there is sluggishness in the performance of her offices, prostration of strength, atony, loss of the faculties of her knees, vertigo, and the limbs sink under her; headache, heaviness of the head, and the woman is pained in the veins on each side of the nose.

But if they fall down, they have heartburn . . . in the hypochondriac regions; flanks empty, where is the seat of the womb; pulse intermittent, irregular, and failing; strong sense of choking; loss of speech and of sensibility; respiration imperceptible and indistinct. . . .

But if the uterus be removed back to its seat before the affection come to a conclusion, they escape the suffocation. When the belly rumbles there is moisture about the female parts, respiration thicker and more distinct, a very speedy rousing up from the affection . . . for as it readily ascends to the higher regions, so it readily recedes. For the uterus is buoyant, but the membranes, its supporters, are humid and the place is humid in which the uterus lies; and, moreover, it flees from fetid things, and seeks after sweet; wherefore, it readily inclines to this side and to that, like a log of wood, and floats upwards and downwards. For this reason the affection occurs in young women, but not in old. For in those in whom the age, mode of life, and understanding is more mobile, the uterus also is of a wandering nature; but in those more advanced in life, the age, mode of living, understanding, and the uterus are of a steady character. Wherefore this suffocation from the womb accompanies females only.

What makes this passage seem even more striking to a modern reader than it already is, is the fact that it was written by a man acclaimed by medical historians for his accuracy in describing the findings in diseases as varied as those we now recognize to have been pneumonia, diabetes, tetanus, elephantiasis, diphtheria, and even bipolar disorder. But in the case of the uterus, all of Aretaeus's skill at observation was to no avail, for there was nothing to observe. The uterus was deep down inside, and he did not dissect the human body.

Though a few of the Cappadocian's predecessors who *had* dissected humans during the glory days of Alexandrian medicine in the third century B.C.E. had demonstrated that the womb is tethered to the depths of the pelvis by stout ligaments, Aretaeus paid them no mind. In this one area of his theoretics he remained in servitude to the ancient powers of rampant imagination, blind to the fact that it was not the uterus that wandered but his own mind. Though the Hippocratics and Galen (who was, as noted earlier, a contemporary of Aretaeus) denied that there was much uterine meandering, they did so in the face of widespread medical and folk confidence that they were wrong. Here, even the hegemony of the great Galen himself was vulnerable. A fourth-century Church incantation has been found in which the uterus is addressed as follows: *Quid irasceris, quid sicut canis iactas te, quid sicut lepus resilis?* ("Why are you mad, why do you throw yourself around like a dog, why do you jump like a hare?")

Though Aretaeus may in the quoted passages have abandoned his usual sobriety of thought, he at least kept the uterus within the confines of the abdominal cavity—he attributed its effects on the voice and the organs of the chest to pressure from below. Earlier commentators and later ones, too, were not so cautious. They wrote of ascents through the thorax and into the voice box. In a later time, Jean Baptiste van Helmont would worry not only about the uterus but about its archeus too. He was convinced that fear of the uterine archeus closed the lung's "pores," thereby causing asthma (which he called epilepsy of the lungs), as well as a long list of other diseases and symptoms, including hysterical contortions of the muscles and joints. The word *hysteria* has in recent decades been formally discarded from the official lexicon of disease terminology, but physicians occasionally still speak of a condition called *globus hystericus,* loosely defined as the sensation of having a lump in one's throat. Few modern doctors know that the lump was originally thought to be the uterus.

Within the past century, the "hysterical" symptom of choking was sometimes alternatively called *suffocatio uterina,* and described in a typical medical dictionary of the late nineteenth century as being "common in hysterical females, and is accompanied with a sensation as if a ball arose from the abdomen to the throat." Parisian physicians of the time called this and related problems *hystérie,* but they were just as likely to refer to it as *ascension de la matrice* or even—perhaps in jest—*mal de mère,* although it was known to those of a more psychiatric bent as *maladie imaginaire.* For good reason, the condition was sometimes configured or conflated with the so-called vapors—which were thought to rise, quite literally, from the womb—and hypochondria, as reflected in yet another diagnosis sometimes made in those days, which must have greatly impressed patients and their families: *hystericohypochondriacum.* But at least no doctor has gone so far afield, literally and figuratively, as certain present-day Silesian and Latvian peasant groups who claim that the uterus can leave the body and travel through forest and meadow. They are not alone in this belief—it has been reported in many other societies at various times and places.

The clinical manifestations of the emotional state that would later become known as hysteria are nowhere better outlined than they are in Aretaeus's description. To him, as to so many physicians and other healers over the centuries, the consequences of the uterus's wanderings constituted a real disease. And quite obviously, "this suffocation from the womb accompanies females alone."

Not only professional healers spoke of hysteria as a definite clinical entity. Like other medical terms, the word came into common use among the laity as well. The most popular self-help book before the twentieth century was William Buchan's *Domestic Medicine.* In many English and American households, the book was exceeded in pride of place only by the Bible; its fervent devotees were facetiously called Buchaneers. My own copy of the 1834 edition is very definite about the symptoms associated with hysteria, although it steers clear of attributing them to a uterine origin. In fact, Buchan specifically refers to the condition as belonging "to the numerous tribe of nervous diseases," and says that it occurs in "[w]omen of a delicate habit, whose stomach and intestines are relaxed, and whose nervous system is extremely sensible," by which he means sensitive. Its characteristics vary in only small details from those pointed out by Aretaeus more than a millennium and a half earlier: he describes swoons, fainting, convulsions, coldness, yawning, stretching, depression, anxiety, laughter, and crying. "At other times the approach of the fit is foretold by a feeling, as if there were a ball at the lower part of the belly, which gradually rises toward the stomach, where it occasions inflation, sickness, and sometimes vomiting; afterwards it rises into the throat, and occasions a fit of suffocation, to which quick breathing, palpitation of the heart, giddiness of the head, dimness of the sight, loss of hearing, with convulsive motions of the extremities and other parts of the body, succeed."

By the time these words were written, any woman who displayed symptoms for which no apparent cause could be identified was fair game to be called a hysterical female, a term that only recently has lost its claim to clinical authenticity. Buchan conveyed the situation in a single sentence: "It appears under such various shapes, imitates so many other diseases, and is attended with such a variety of symptoms, that it is difficult to give a just character or definition of it; and it is only by taking the aggregate of its appearances that a proper idea can be conveyed of it to others."

Buchan pointed out a characteristic of hysteria that has baffled clinicians again and again, and still does, namely its occasional "contagiousness." Epidemics of its symptoms have taken many forms, but none more spellbinding—and I use the word deliberately—than those involving the so-called incubus. Incubi were said to be male demons who had their way with innocent young women, including more than a few nuns. The maraudings of the ectoplasmic satyrs were reported frequently during the Middle Ages and Renaissance, and occasionally an outbreak occurred in a particular locality. Innocent VIII, who was pope from 1484 to 1492, believed so strongly in witchcraft that he not only dispatched inquisitors to root it out (the most prominent of whom were the aforementioned Kramer and Sprenger), but issued a bull in which was contained a formula for exorcising an incubus or its female equivalent, the far less prevalent succubus.

The author of *Domestic Medicine* also noted a characteristic of epidemic hysteria that has not infrequently been found useful in the treatment of afflicted patients—the use of suggestion in those patients in whom suggestion may have played a role in initiating the symptoms in the first place: "When hysteric fits are occasioned by sympathy, they may be cured by exciting an opposite passion. This is said to have been the case of a whole school of young ladies in Holland, who were all cured by being told, that the first who was seized should be burned to death. But this method of cure, to my knowledge, will not always succeed. I would therefore advise, that young ladies who are subject to hysteric fits, should not be sent to boarding-schools, as the disease may be caught by imitation."

Buchan may not have been among them, but in his time general medical opinion continued to relate hysteria to the uterus. (In addition, there were some late nineteenth-century physicians who attributed hysterical symptoms to the ovaries, going so far as to call the disease *oophoria*.) The notion would persist until relatively modern times. Although the conceit of "wandering" gradually disappeared, physicians maintained their belief in the condition's uterine origin well beyond the point at which simple observation should have convinced them that a patient required no *hystera* to be hysterical—the selfsame symptoms could be found in men.

Not until approximately the turn of the seventeenth century was it so much as suggested that the cause of hysteria should be sought not in the uterus but in the brain. This innovative idea was first put forth by Charles Lepois, physician to King Henry II of France, but he was ignored. So closely associated with the female disposition (and indisposition) did hysteria long remain that the young Sigmund Freud was ridiculed when he returned to Vienna in 1886 from his period of study in Paris, for pointing out what he called "the frequent occurrence of hysteria in men." In his *Autobiographical Study,* Freud quotes an elderly Viennese surgeon who actually said to him, "But, my dear sir, how can you talk such nonsense? *Hysteron* [*sic*] means the uterus. So how can a man be hysterical?"

At the time of Freud's experience, Vienna was one of the most advanced of the citadel-cities of medicine, and yet the realization that hysteria required no *hystera* had not yet entered medical thought, though it was beginning to be widely accepted elsewhere. America's leading gynecologist of the period, Charles Meigs of the Jefferson Medical College in Philadelphia, had stated the fact clearly in his 1851 book, *Woman: Her Diseases and Remedies.* But as he also reminded his readers, the old notion of an object or force rising from below had not completely disappeared, at least among the laity. Meigs writes of a young Irish immigrant woman who came to him in 1843 with a problem she called the wandering arrow, because, in the words of her mother, "Why, it begins at the bottom of her stomach, sir, and it goes winding up along the course of her bowels until it gets to her throat, and then it chokes her, and she has a fit."

With a vast clinical experience on which to draw, Meigs was convinced that hysteria was a manifestation of what he called the aphrodisiac force, in other words, that there was an element in the patient's sexual drive that caused it. It was his conviction that those medical writers who still persisted in associating hysteria with the womb were, whether knowingly or not, speaking not of the womb itself but of the whole genital apparatus from which sexual passion was thought to arise. They were thus displacing what they believed to be sexually charged emotional content onto an organ they reasoned to be associated with sexuality. This is in effect a fascinatingly prescient—even if unknowing—analogy with the real etiology of hysteria, which is thought to be a conversion of a morbid thought pattern into physical symptoms or behavior. Early thinkers seem to have focused on the womb in an attempt to attach a location to their incompletely formed perception that hysterical symptoms may have a psychosexual meaning.

Meigs's is a particularly suggestive observation because it reflects a theme that seems to have been woven irregularly into medical thought from antiquity to the present. As early as the Hippocratic writings, there can be found the recommendation that marriage is the best remedy for these sorts of symptoms: "For hysterical maidens, I prescribe marriage, for they are cured by pregnancy." This echoes the notions of Plato's *Timaeus* quoted earlier, a book written during the lifetime of Hippocrates. Although the Egyptians and others had made vague allusions to it, it was in the Hippocratic writings, in fact, that the first recorded suggestion appears that the catalog of otherwise unexplainable symptoms was the result of some abnormal uterine condition.

From the very beginning of the Hippocratic period, there appear repeated references that unrequited sexual desire is in some way the culprit. Sexual frustration, in fact, was thought by some to be one of the causes of uterine leapings. But not all of the ancient physicians were convinced of the relationship between hysteria and the peripatetic womb. Writing in the first half of the second century C.E., Soranus of Ephesus, the Roman Empire's leading authority on gynecology, went so far as to deny any significant movement to the uterus, even when it was sick: "For the uterus does not issue forth like a wild animal from the lair, delighted by fragrant odors and fleeing bad odors; rather [in cases of hysteria] it is drawn together because of stricture caused by inflammation." To Soranus, hysteria was the product of an inflammatory process that resulted in constriction and retraction of the uterus. So opposed to Hippocratic thinking was he on the subject that Soranus interdicted sexual intercourse as a treatment. Treatment demanded strengthening, he said, and sexual activity accomplishes just the opposite: "Intercourse causes atony in everybody and is therefore not appropriate."

Galen was among those who doubted that the uterus was capable of much migration, but he nevertheless concurred with his Hippocratic predecessors that sexual frustration was a prominent cause of hysteria. He taught that hysteria is the result of congestion of the uterus rather than wanderings of the organ, and was known to advise treatment by manual stimulation of the clitoris or uterine cervix. He believed the uterine engorgement to be sometimes caused by retention of the menses, but more commonly by what he called accumulation of semen (in the ancient world, the word *semen* was used in this way, to denote a nonspecific fluid that was believed to be the female equivalent of the male ejaculate) due to lack of sexual intercourse. The retained semen was said to become "badly composed," and to continue to cause symptoms until it was discharged from the body. In his tract "The Affected Parts," Galen describes a patient of whom he had been informed, who was afflicted with what he calls nervous tension. A midwife had told her that the condition was due to the womb having become displaced upward, and recommended a medication which, by causing warmth, was meant to bring the wandering organ back down to its proper position: "On application, the heat of this medicine and the contact with her sexual organs provoked [uterine] contractions associated with the pain and pleasure similar to that experienced during intercourse. As result the woman secreted a large quantity of heavy semen and thus lost the bothersome complaints."

Soranus was highly regarded and often quoted, but in other ancient, medieval, and Renaissance writings, evidence appears from time to time that—like Galen—one or another observer has wittingly or unwittingly perceived a psychosexual context to the symptoms of hysteria. The implication—and in some cases the certainty—runs like a constantly recurring theme through the works of a series of authors. And the notion of the wandering womb would simply not go away. Ambroise Paré, the greatest of the Renaissance surgeons, recommended that the vagina of a suffering patient be held open by a gold or silver dilator, so that "sweet and aromaticke fumigations" might waft their way upward toward the womb, from a specially constructed metal vessel placed between the woman's legs, under which a fire was lit. The long-necked vessel was to contain a mixture of cinnamon, lavender, benzoin, pennyroyal, calomine, nutmeg, musk, "and such like, which for their sweet smell and sympathy, allure or entice the wombe downewards, by their heat consume and digest the thicke vapours, and putrefied ill juice." Not content with this alone, he advised also "that a great cupping-glasse with a great flame be applyed to the belly below the navell, to the inner part of the thigh, and to the groin, whereby the matter that climes upwards, and also the womb it self running the same way, may be brought downwards or drawn back." By these several means, Paré was treating the wandering womb and its ascending vapors. The digestion of the "putrefied ill juice" was meant to consume Galen's "accumulation of semen." Paré was one of the many who attributed hysteria to what he called "suppression of their seede."

But Paré was not yet through; there was another factor to consider if the problem was to be attacked on all fronts and with all possibilities in mind: "[I]f she be married, let her forthwith use copulation, and bee strongly encountered by her husband, for there is no remedy more present than this." And there was additional advice, presumably for those without husbands. In this case, the midwife was to anoint her finger with oil into which had been stirred a mixture of various sweet powders, "and let her rub or tickle the top of the necke of the wombe which toucheth the inner orifice; but her secret parts must first be warmed by the applying of warme linnen clothes, for so at length the venomous matter contained in the wombe, shall bee dissolved and flow out, and the maligne, sharpe and flatulent vapours, whereby the wombe is driven as it were into a fury or rage, shall bee resolved and dissipated, and so when the conjunct matter of the disease is scattered and wasted, the wombe, and also the woman shall bee restored unto themselves again."

Paracelsus, Paré's contemporary, in whose tortuous writings a vein of gold is sometimes struck where least expected, without further explanation suggested the name *chorea lasciva* for the seizurelike movements that in his time were lumped under the general title of St. Vitus' dance. Nowadays, St. Vitus' dance is considered a symptom of rheumatic fever, and is known to be accompanied by a degree of emotional instability. But in the time of Paracelsus, the name was applied to a wide variety of uncoordinated involuntary movements like those exhibited in some hysterical patients. He blamed the disease on the imagination, claiming that adults exhibit the movements because they have seen and remembered them (which recalls Buchan's statement about imitation, although in a different context), whereas in children, "unconsciously they have fantasies about what they have seen and heard. And in such fantasies their reason is taken and perverted into the shape imagined." This appears to be the first overt recognition ever recorded of the conversion of an emotional or unconscious state into physical manifestations, which is now known to be a prominent factor in the syndrome that has been called hysteria. That Paracelsus, renowned as a woman-hater, would attach the

word *lasciva* to it, suggests that he more than suspected sexual connotations.

In the seventeenth century, the term *Sydenham's chorea* began to be
applied to the contorted movements of St. Vitus' dance when they appeared in children between approximately the age of ten and puberty.
This was the beginning of the process of narrowing down by which we
today associate the symptom with rheumatic fever. It acquired that
name because it was originally described by the prominent English clinician Thomas Sydenham. Interestingly, Sydenham, too, appears to
have intuited a possible causative relationship between hysteria and
matters psychosexual.

Thomas Sydenham was a man without patience for experiment or
theory. It is said that he knew little and cared less about the great
anatomical contributions of Andreas Vesalius or the physiological descriptions of William Harvey. His household god was Hippocrates, and
like the Hippocratic physicians, all of his emphasis was on his own experiences at the bedside. In an aphoristic moment, he summoned up
his philosophy as follows: "The art of medicine is to be properly
learned only from its practice and exercise." He was a masterful observer and an outstanding example of a man endowed with the quality that modern physicians admiringly call clinical intuition, earned
less through an encyclopedic command of textbook facts than by a
combination of the stored wisdom attained through accumulated encounters with disease, keen perception of observed phenomena, a
good ear for listening, powerful intellect, and good judgment.

Included in Sydenham's collected works is a short article entitled
"Of the disorder which is called hysteric passion in women, and the
hypochondriac disease in men." Although, like so many others of the
time, he conflated the two conditions, it is clear from a reading of the
text that the greater part of his attention is paid to that multiplicity of
symptoms most commonly associated with hysteria: "Simply to enu-
merate all the symptoms of hysteria would take a long day, so many
are they. Yet not more numerous than varied, proteoform, and
chameleonlike."

Sydenham recommends that treatment of the illness be started with a bleeding of eight ounces and the application of a plaster to the navel, permeated with galbanum, a bitter gum resin. On the following morning, a series of medicines is begun, consisting of assorted mixtures of some of the standards of the day, such as Peruvian balsam, wormwood, iron filings, nutmeg, certain fruit particles, coriander, anise, wake-robin, gentian water, clove-july flowers, myrrh, turpentine, amber, hartshorn, laudanum, and a variety of purgatives. After presenting a series of nineteen numbered paragraphs outlining the proper sequence of therapeutic regimens, Sydenham reaches the final sentence of the article: "But nothing does so effectually strengthen the blood, and raise the spirits, as riding much on horse-back almost every day for a considerable time; and riding in a coach is no contemptible remedy."

Historians of psychiatry point to this ultimate bit of advice as evidence that Sydenham on some level understood the symbolic significance of hysteria, and perhaps of horseback riding too. Although one should be wary of making too much of the connection (especially in view of horseback riding as general therapy having long been recommended by many physicians), the horse is associated in the psychoanalytic literature with the phallus. If this formulation is valid, then the master clinician perceived or intuited that a sublimated sexual need can be treated by a sublimated sexual release.

Of course, the release may not always be as sublimated as one might think. In the hands—literally—of some doctors, genital massage to orgasm seems for centuries to have been one of the accepted treatments for hysteria, whether by the physician, a female attendant, or the patient herself. Paré was hardly alone among the different kinds of healers who describe one or another variation of it. It is obvious that considerations of the condition's relationship to Galen's "accumulation of semen" not only persisted but with the passage of time became widely accepted. Around the turn of the twentieth century, external genital vibrators and the rocking motion of specially designed "jolting chairs" were sometimes being used in the treatment of women suffering from a group of conditions (seen in both sexes) falling under the general heading of what physicians called neurasthenia, among which hysteria was included. A neurasthenic patient, whether male or female, suffered with what William Osler's authoritative 1892 textbook of medicine described as "a condition of weakness or exhaustion of the nervous system." The term "covers an ill-defined, motley group of symptoms" which produce effects that might be neurological, cardiac, gastric, sexual, or generalized. The fact that Osler devoted twelve pages to his discussion of hysteria indicates how significant the disease was thought to be at the time. His general recommendations for treatment are based on the principles of "isolation, rest, diet, massage, and electricity," the latter two modalities to be applied—thankfully—not to the genitals but to the voluntary muscles of the body.

When the eighth edition of his text appeared in 1919, Osler had added psychotherapy and the consideration of hypnosis to the proposed regimen. By then, such was the growing authority of Sigmund Freud's pioneering work in the psychoanalytic treatment of hysteria that Osler devoted almost two full pages to a discussion of the Viennese technique (which he calls "in reality the old method of the confessional, in which the sinner poured out his soul in the sympathetic ear of the priest"). The major point of Freud's theory of hysteria was that it originated in repressed memories of fantasized or real seduction during childhood. He hypothesized that the patient's need to prevent resurfacing of the memory caused the sexual drive to be converted into a specific physical symptom, whose function was to relieve the fear that the patient would yield to unacceptable sexual impulses. The symptom was said to be symbolic of the action that was feared. This theory provided the basic structure for the modern treatment of hysteria and its related conditions. Today, of course, the psychosexual basis of hysteria—male and female—is a staple of psychoanalytic theory.

But not under the name of hysteria. That word has recently been abandoned in response to the realities of the condition and the justified protests of women in general and feminists in particular. Now known as conversion reaction, hysteria is diagnosed in certain situations when symptoms exist suggesting a physical disorder that cannot be confirmed by objective findings—whether in males or females.

The Diagnostic and Statistical Manual of the American Psychiatric Association for 1979 (DSM-III) still listed "hysterical neurosis," but DSM-IV of 1994 refers to "conversion reactions."

This is not to imply that the terms *hysteria* and *hysterical female* never pass the lips of physicians and others, but they are no longer recognized as clinical conditions. In fact, both terms are condemned as pejoratives, although most physicians practicing today were trained in an era when the terms were not only commonplace but accepted as medical entities. An example of the prevalence of the image of the hysterical female is to be found in a well-remembered informational booklet distributed to American doctors by the Ciba-Geigy Corporation. The *Ciba Clinical Symposia* have been highly regarded by several generations of physicians for their reliable and thorough descriptions of disease entities, accompanied by illustrations so accurate and artistic that they have become widely known and reproduced for a variety of educational purposes. A thirty-four-page issue of 1977 entitled "Hysteria: A Clinical Guide to Diagnosis" bears on its front cover a colorful drawing of a fortyish blonde whose fashionably slim body is tucked at a provocative angle into an orange armchair, one hand resting high on her lap as though modestly to cover her pubis. The other trails a lit cigarette held lightly between her delicately extended fingers. She is stylishly and even suggestively attired in leather boots, a short skirt, and a tight sweater. A coy smile brightens the visage she has turned toward her doctor in an obvious attempt to charm. Holding her hair in place is an encircling black band, held tight around her head by a small, winchlike structure affixed behind her left ear. She is at once sexually inviting and evidently disturbed.

Although therapy based on psychoanalytic principles continues to be used extensively to treat symptoms falling into the general category of the condition traditionally known as hysteria, other of the older remedies, whether for hysteria or other uterus-related problems, have long since been consigned to the annals of unrepeatable history. Still, some of them did endure for centuries and even millennia before they faded into oblivion. When Aretaeus made his recommendation that hysterical suffocation be treated by "fetid smells, and the application of fragrant things to the female parts," such advice was already old. Its earliest written description is to be found in Egyptian papyri, but the concept must have long preceded that civilization. The treatment is based on the idea that since "the womb is an animal within an animal," it should be attracted by pleasant odors and repelled by unpleasant ones. If this was true, its sense of smell could be used to return it to its pelvic position when it strayed.

A practical application of this theory was its use in the Egyptian treatment of prolapse, or dropped uterus, a condition not uncommon in those days of multiple births and relative ignorance of obstetric physiology. The Ebers papyrus describes an incense made of dried human excrement, with the instructions, "The woman bends herself over the same and lets the fumes thereof penetrate into her sex organs," no doubt in the hope that the stench will drive the womb upward to its proper position.

Likewise, the inhalation of pleasant fragrances was also meant to encourage the womb to rise to its normal position. There is no record of the results of these olfactory methods, but we do know that the Egyptians supplemented them with mechanical means, such as the pressure of a finger in the vagina, anointed with honey and oils, "a remedy to enable the uterus of woman to return to its proper region," as the Ebers papyrus describes it. The Hippocratics, who were familiar with the use of pessaries, devices inserted into the vagina to support or reposition the uterus, were known to support a dropped womb by inserting half a pomegranate as high as possible into the vagina, having previously soaked the fruit in lukewarm wine.

Like so many other civilizations, the Egyptians blamed all sorts of "female" problems on the erratic behavior of the womb. The Kahun papyrus of the third millennium B.C.E., devoted to gynecologic and veterinary matters, lists an entire catalog of pains traceable to the much-maligned organ—of the neck, eye sockets, limbs, belly, and ears. Moreover, if a woman "loves the bed [and] she does not rise," it is due to "grasping of the womb." Ascent of the uterus is elsewhere in the papyrus said to be the cause of certain eye and throat disorders.

For such indispositions, a variety of treatments is offered: the vulva may be perfumed by incense and anointed with fresh oil; one should pour on the woman the urine of an ass that has engendered two colts on the day of the pain, in this case urinary burning; rub her feet; or have her drink a mixture of corn and beer on four consecutive mornings. Such implausible treatments are found in the midst of others that, by their nature, must have been effective. Among them are the insertion of pessaries consisting of a ball of lint or flax soaked in any of a variety of herbal preparations.

Prayer, of course, has always played a very important role in the treatment of disease of any nature, accompanied by a wide range of the varieties of sacrifice, charity, and charms. Because so-called women's diseases have been so prevalent and attributed to magical causes, particularly in early societies, a long tradition exists of what might be called extra-medical aids to recovery. Prominent among them are images of female organs, serving as votive objects.

If the word *votive* is defined as referring to the expression of a vow or a wish, then it is obvious why such objects have long been associated with prayers for healing the sick. Although there is no evidence that votive objects existed in Egypt, they have been found in large numbers at various European sites representing a wide range of historical periods. For example, in a temple to Amyto, an early Greek god of healing who precedes even Aesculapius (which would place him before approximately 1000 B.C.E.), a terra-cotta leg with varicose veins has been discovered. Similar images in metal and stone have been dug up elsewhere, often depicting body parts like a rough-hewn limb or an open abdomen or chest with the coarse representations of the viscera within, or at least those thought to be the origin of the sickness. Facial parts, hands, feet, and skeletal structures have also been found, intended to beseech or propitiate one or another god. In various areas of the world, folk or peasant societies still turn to votive articles of metal, wax, stone, wood, or terra-cotta as part of the process of seeking cure.

Female generative organs have always been featured among the most prominent of the votive objects, their powers being commonly invoked to assure sexual fulfillment and successful reproduction. Whether to ward off the spells of witches and sprites or to aid in generating healthy offspring, models of labia, uteri, and even the placenta were brought to the ancient temples to fructify a union and enhance sexual performance. They were also used to petition for a safer delivery or to give thanks for recovery from disease or a difficult labor. Representations of breasts were meant to aid in lactation. In Greece and Rome, bakers made little cakes in the form of the genitals of both sexes, to be sacrificed to such gods as Priapus and Venus.

But even in this, the uterus was unique. It appears to be the only organ represented in votive imagery by an animal. The animal is the toad. Although it might be thought that this is because a vague similarity in appearance exists between a womb and a plump toad, it is far more likely that the custom derives directly from the notion of the organ's animatistic nature and its leaping peregrinations from place to place. The toad has always been considered a powerful symbol in the lore of magic, mystically known in German as a *Seelentier,* or "soul animal." It is not too far-fetched to wonder whether this too may derive from the uterus. I have even seen a photograph of a modern toad votive bearing on its back an artistically etched cross, as though to illustrate the fuzzy border that lies between the fringes of religious practice and the encroachments of superstition. Whether the uterus or any other structure of the body is being studied, medical lore is replete with examples of the human inability to separate faith from confabulation and fact from fantasy.

The great joined triumvirate of superstition, religion, and science has remained a powerful force in the individual philosophies of the people of our time. The three have been so tightly interwoven that the thought processes of the great mass of men and women are assaulted by a plethora of stimuli coming now from one, now from another—and sometimes the sources are indistinguishable; even the most determined minds find them difficult to separate. The rules of evidence are laid aside, as the rules of passion, wishful thinking, and faith intrude on what should be the detached pursuit of verifiable knowledge. The dilemma has ever been with us and will ever be.

Though it no longer impedes the progress of science to the extent it did in the past, the confusing triple admixture has long held a grip on the human mind. It may loosen with more time, but we will never be free from it.

The following chapter tells the story of what is perhaps the most blatant example of an aspect of discovery in which the interrelationships among the three strange bedfellows produced strange offspring.

CHAPTER TEN

REPRODUCTION:

BABIES IN BOXES

I F the uterus itself mystified, its functions in menstruation and re-production must have absolutely confounded the minds of even the most dispassionate thinkers of the prescientific period. The combination of the bleeding and its sometimes unpredictable perio-dicity added layers to the organ's reputation for autonomous and will-ful behavior. For several days of each month, a copious quantity of the source of life itself was discharged through a woman's vagina, and yet she seemed neither weakened by its loss nor permanently affected by the mood swings that sometimes precede the period of menses. In some traditions, the catamenia, or menstrual flow, was thought to contain a powerful force for evil, and in others an equally powerful force for good. Some were certain, for example, that a menstruating woman's mere presence would destroy the fruits of the field and cor-rode metal; others insisted that menstrual blood has healing effects when used properly. It was rare to encounter someone who had no opinion about its good or bad qualities, far more commonly the latter.

The Church and the Synagogue concurred. Leviticus, 15:19 states, "And if a woman have an issue, and her issue in her flesh be blood, she shall be put apart seven days: and whosoever toucheth her shall be unclean until the even." Based on this biblical passage Jews considered a woman impure during her menses, requiring that she visit the *mikveh,* or ritual bath, at an appropriate time after their conclusion, in order to be cleansed. "The husband in that period should not touch her even with his little finger," proclaims the *Shulhan Arukh,* the great code of Jewish law promulgated in the sixteenth century and to this day the revered guidebook of the Orthodox. She may enter the synagogue only on the ten Days of Awe, from the New Year until the Day of Atonement, although special permission is granted when her son or daughter is married or if she has just given birth and is still passing blood.

In a letter written in 247 C.E., carrying the force of canon law, Dionysius, the Archbishop of Alexandria, made the position of the Church very clear: "Menstruous women ought not to come to the Holy Table, or touch the Holy of Holies [in the original Greek, this is "the body and blood of Christ"], nor to churches, but pray elsewhere." Bishop Isidore of Seville, the author of an encyclopedia containing a survey of medicine and said to be the most learned man of the seventh century, had this to say of menstrual blood: "On contact with this gore, crops do not generate, wine goes sour, trees lose their fruit, iron is corrupted by rust, copper is blackened. Should dogs eat any of it they go mad. Even bituminous glue which is dissolved neither by rain nor by strong water, polluted by this gore, falls apart by itself."

Whether its issue was impure or not, the uterus was obviously an organ in which life is generated. But how can life be nurtured by the same structure that regularly bleeds and thereby casts life out? Not only that question required an answer but so did the mystery of why the monthly flow ceases when a new life is beginning to form and does not resume until well after the infant has left the womb. Early writers on these matters can hardly be blamed for concluding that the retained blood must in some way take part in the process by which procreation occurs. The most prevalent theory had menstrual blood being clotted by the addition of the male seed—an undefined substance carried in the semen—to produce the material of the embryo.

Some of the writings of the golden age of Greece in the fifth and fourth centuries B.C.E. describe the process of fertilization to be analogous to the clotting of milk by an activating substance. There are plenty of precedents for such an idea, including a reference in the Book of Job, written around 500 B.C.E. In a speech he plans to make to God, Job says, "Hast thou not poured me out as milk, and curdled me like cheese?" (10:10).

Several prominent Greek thinkers promoted the notion that the activator of the coagulation process is the semen of the male. Others claimed that the child exists preformed in the semen, which uses the clumped blood only as a source of nourishment much as a seed implants itself in fertile soil. This last was a concept inherited directly from the Egyptians.

The Egyptians believed that the semen—which in their writings appears to be identical to the seed—originates in the spinal cord and passes directly from there into the testicles. The function of the lowermost vertebrae, which are fused into a single bone, was thought to be the protection of the semen's source. Because the thick, solid structure was therefore considered to have a mystical purpose, it became known as the sacred bone, and in later languages the sacrum.

Semen was believed by the Egyptians to originate not only in the spinal cord but in the heart too. From there, it was said to be transported via the *metu* to the testicles. One text describes how the "man laid his heart in the woman," but the Egyptians, while recognizing the importance of the placenta, seem not to have otherwise described any maternal contribution to the fetus.

In all ancient writings, the nature of the seed was itself problematic. What, specifically, was it?* Was it identical to semen? Where does it come from? What does it contain? How does it contribute to the characteristics of the embryo? It is to be expected that the notion of seed, being the germinal source of the embryo and the primary substance from which the new life arises, would be confused with semen, the male ejaculate. But they were not necessarily the same thing, and in any case it was hardly certain that seed came only from the male. Some

---

*Predictably, van Helmont would regard it as a "spiritual gas" having a foreknowledge of what it must do.

believed that a woman's nonmenstrual vaginal fluids were also semen, or perhaps seed. Since there was no universal agreement on these matters, what was the seed's place of origin? Some said that it came from the whole body, some said the testicles, some the vaginal secretions, others the brain, spinal cord, or spinal marrow. The Hippocratic writings, although somewhat internally contradictory, in general leave the impression that the seed comes from the whole body, including its fluids.

Theories maintaining that the seed comes exclusively from the menstrual blood and those identifying its origin in the semen could not explain why the offspring seemed to share the features of both parents, or more confusing yet, sometimes resemble mostly the one not credited with being the source. Empedocles attempted to solve this problem by theorizing that each parent contributed seed in which was housed a preformed individual. Parts from each were said to be torn loose and fitted to one another in the womb. (He was prescient. Nowadays we know that an exchange, or crossing over, of small amounts of DNA occurs between the father's member of the matched chromosome pair and the mother's, resulting in a genetic recombination that amounts to what is essentially new DNA containing genes from both parents.)

Another riddle was how to account for the sex of the offspring. A popular Hippocratic belief attributed it to whichever testicle was the source of the semen: the right was said to produce males and the left females. In the text *Superfetation,* one of the Hippocratic writers goes so far as to suggest that the sex of the offspring be controlled by tying off one testicle. But the general Hippocratic view was nevertheless that each parent contributes what was called an active and a material principle to the formation of the embryo. The active principle provided the energy to make the process of generation take place; the material provided the matter from which the child was made. In this view, not only was the substance of the child derived from both mother and father, but so was its activating energy.

Aristotle's theory of generation was developed from several sources: the notions of his predecessors; his systematic studies of sequential chick embryos and embryos of other animals; and his own ideas about living things in general. In his formulation, the female of the species provides the egg (or in menstruating animals, the catamenia) containing the ingredients of what will be the eventual embryo. The male's semen provides the source of the activity—the activating force—but not any of the actual matter from which the embryo is produced. In humans, therefore: "When the material secreted by the female in the uterus has been fixed by the semen of the male (this acts in the same way as rennet acts upon milk, for rennet is a kind of milk containing vital heat, which brings into one mass and fixes the similar material, and the relation of the semen to the catamenia is the same, milk and the catamenia being of the same nature), when, I say, the more solid part comes together, the liquid is separated off from it, and as the earthy parts solidify membranes form all around it."

It was Aristotle's contention that a new activity or energy is started up by the coming together of semen and egg (or catamenia), which continues as long as the generated individual lives. He further asserted that all seed, male and female, comes eventually from the blood. The seed is therefore among the ultimate results of the process of digestion, by which the blood is manufactured in the liver.

If the great Greek naturalist believed that the male semen comes from the blood, what did he conceive to be the function of the testicles? Ever the innovative thinker, he said that they act as weights, to tighten and presumably straighten the passages through which the semen flows. To his credit, though, he does describe a process of compaction that takes place in the testicles, by which the semen is concentrated to its final viscosity.

Briefly then, Aristotle taught that the contributions of the two parents are complementary to each other. It was his view that the generative principle—the force that makes everything happen—resides in the male semen. The female semen (read menstrual blood), on the other hand, was said to provide the nutritive and material expression of the fetus, whose form is determined by the generative force contributed by the male.

Predictably, Galen would have his own views. He accepted the Hippocratic idea that the right testicle makes males and the left females, but he also agreed with some of his predecessors that the equivalent sides of the womb have the same effect. He based these notions on the theory of humors: the right side is closer to the warm, moist liver, while the left is under the cold, dry, spleen.

Galen had the advantage over Aristotle of knowing of the existence of ovaries, because they had been discovered by Herophilus, one of the Alexandrian physicians who dissected human bodies in the third century B.C.E. Galen was convinced that testicles serve as reservoirs for semen, whose source he believed to be the entire body. He rejected the thesis that the menstrual blood plays any role in the formation of the embryo. He pictured the series of necessary events as follows: During intercourse, the cervix opens wide to allow the male seed or semen to enter the uterus. At the same time, the female seed or semen is discharged from its reservoir in the ovaries and mixes with its male counterpart (Galen's evidence for the existence of female semen was the presence of fluid in the vagina during sexual arousal. His formulation amounted to the suggestion that both males and females ejaculate at the time of coitus). At this point, the uterus contracts around the mixture of the two semens in order to hold it in, and the cervix closes tightly. The contraction spreads the mixture over the rough inner lining of the uterus to form a thin membrane, acted upon by the combined pneuma of its two components. Generation begins from this membrane and leads to the eventual development of the three organs considered by Galen to be the sources of all other structures in the body and of life itself—the liver, the heart, and the brain. Galen argued that the entire embryo arises in one way or another from the rudiments of these three. He taught that the reproductive apparatus is in some way connected to each member of the trio, in order to draw the constituents of male or female from them. By way of typical Galenic teleology, he goes on to say: "Nature had three principal aims in constructing the parts of the animal; for she made them either for the sake of life (the brain, heart and liver), or for a better life (the eyes, ears and nostrils) or for the continuance of the race (the pudenda, testes and uteri)." It should not be overlooked that in writing of the womb, Galen customarily used the plural "uteri." Being unfamiliar with human anatomy, he was referring to the two horn-shaped branches that characterize the uterus of most mammals. He was certain that a woman's anatomy was the same.

Whatever its defects, Galen's formulation was based on his recognition that both male and female contribute more or less equally to the eventual offspring. In spite of his profound influence over subsequent medical theory, later authors seem not to have bought into this conception of conception. Confused and confusing theories persisted all through the Middle Ages, containing various elements of Greek thought and attempts at its emendation.

In the sphere of comprehending reproduction, as in so many others, progress appears linear only if the many points above and below the seemingly smooth upward slope are erased or ignored. One of the most out-of-range dots on the graph of reproductive enlightenment—*the* most distant, in fact—was put into place by that mercurial genius Paracelsus, he of the enormous leaps of inspired thought that were now insightful and now wildly fallacious. The following outright confabulation is to be found in Book I of his *Treatise Concerning the Nature of Things:*

> Let the sperm of a man by itself be putrefied in a gourd glass, sealed up, with the highest degree of putrefaction in horse-dung, for the space of forty days, or so long until it begin to be alive, move, and stir, which may easily be seen. After this time it will be something like a man, yet transparent, and without a body. Now after this, if it be every day warily, and prudently nourished and fed with the arcanum* of man's blood, and be for the space of forty weeks kept in a constant, equal heat of horse-dung, it will become a true, and living infant, having all the members of an infant, which is born of a woman, but it will be far less. This we call *Homunculus*† or artificial man. . . . Now this is one of the greatest secrets, that God ever made known to mortal, sinful man.

---

*This word reflects the influence of alchemy on Paracelsus's thinking. Arcanum is Latin for "secret." In the alchemists' terminology, it refers to the ultimate secret of nature, which they strove to discover.

†Note that homunculus *as used here refers to an artificial man. In more common usage, the word refers simply to a miniature man. This is the way it would be used by later authors who believed that each person is preformed in the father's sperm or the mother's egg.*

No wonder that Michel de Montaigne, commenting in the middle of the sixteenth century on the contemporary he refers to as "some newcomer called Paracelsus," says of him, " 'Believe nobody,' as the saying goes. 'Anyone can *say* anything'" [italics in original].

The "anything" of Paracelsus is well beyond reason. Still, it shines a light, however dim, on the vast spectrum of unsuspected influences that affect any investigator's understanding of surroundings and of self. It need hardly be reiterated that throughout the history of mankind's study of nature, interpretations of observed phenomena have been determined by powerful elements in the *zeitgeist,* the spirit of the time. Theological, philosophical, social, and even political considerations have been the lenses through which the findings and offerings of the scientist have been viewed, even by the scientists themselves—beyond those which are personal and related to an individual's own psychological structure. Still now at the turn of the twenty-first century, many scientists have difficulty accepting that certain innate biases influence, no matter how subtly, their interpretation of any observed occurrence, not to say their use of it and the way in which they fit it into their general perception of nature. Whether in the form of an era's great scientific paradigms (as the philosopher of science Thomas Kuhn has proposed), or as minuscule personal particularities and dispositions, no researcher can be completely free of taint in this regard. The most thoughtful of investigators recognize this and try to identify the ways in which they may properly accuse themselves of lacking dispassion, in order to root them out as far as is possible; lesser men and women work on, blissfully ignorant or uncaring of their effects.

It is so easy to identify and smugly condemn those now-obvious defects of reasoning as we look backward over the centuries. Immersed in their unique time and its philosophy as they are, the researchers and thinkers of any era can rarely see high enough or far enough— even when they actually look—to recognize their own culpability. Even those who can, have difficulty knowing what to do about it. And so, the greatest minds of every generation inevitably leave a heritage of imperfections in the midst of their finest achievements. We can only wonder how our own errors will be unearthed and perceived by future generations.

One need not be a radical feminist to appreciate that one of the most flagrant sources of error in the interpretation not only of biological events but of the findings of other disciplines, too, has been the tacit assumption of women's less than significant role in the course of natural events. Man molded from the very essence of the earth itself cannot be equaled by woman molded from his rib. Her life came from him. God "breathed into his nostrils the breath of life," as we read in Genesis. Thus, even the first pneuma, or the first spirit, was man's and not woman's. Her life came from him. St. Augustine states it even more starkly in his *City of God* (XII, 21): "God created only one single man . . . and indeed He did not even create the woman that was to be given him as his wife, as he created the man, but created her out of the man, that the whole human race might derive from one man." Her life came from him. Gregory the Great, remembered as the social liberalizer who transformed the papacy during his fourteen-year pontificate (590–604) and was responsible for the chants that bear his name, taught that Eve was only flesh, whereas Adam was mind and spirit. Her life came from him.

We have inherited a culture permeated with the assumption of the subordinate position of women. Sometimes the traditional inequity descends into misogyny.

Misogyny characterizes the statement of Paracelsus quoted a few pages back. Every man has met such men, who are less likely to reveal themselves to women. Apparently repelled (likely terrified, as a psychoanalyst might put it) by female anatomy and function, Paracelsus convinced himself that all reproduction is in some way dependent upon putrefaction. This is in accord with the belief that menstrual blood—since earliest times widely thought to be a source of contamination—is the nourishing substance for the embryo. To prove his contention, he described the "experiment" (which he could not possibly have succeeded in completing) in which an artificial man is generated from sperm and horse dung. The dung has replaced the traditional catamenia. Ergo, menstrual blood and dung are equivalent; ergo a woman's role can be filled by dung. Here we have the thinking behind the feminist slogan "A woman needs a man like a fish needs a bicycle" turned on its head centuries before it existed. Fortunately, this particular flight of Paracelsian fancy seems to have been ignored even by that imaginative thinker's most committed disciples.

Of the several theories of human reproduction that *were* taken seriously during Paracelsus's time, there was one that would come to permeate the beliefs of the theologians, the laity, and even some scientists until almost two centuries ago. This was the idea that each individual is already preformed in the seed of one or the other of its parents. To many churchmen, this was implied in the words of St. Augustine, "that the whole human race might derive from one man," but it had earlier found unequivocal expression in a statement in Seneca's *Quaestiones naturales* of the first century C.E.:

> In the seed are enclosed all the parts of the body of the man that shall be formed. The infant that is borne in his mother's wombe hath the rootes of the beard and hair that he shall weare one day. In this little masse likewise are all the lineaments of the bodie and all that which Posterity shall discover in him.

Empedocles, Plato, and the early fathers of the Church subscribed to this notion, which in a later era would be called the theory of preformation. Not surprisingly, the early preformationists were certain that the uterus is only the soil in which the seed grows and that sex is determined by the side upon which the seed falls into the menstrual blood. The preformation theory made sense to Christians because it meant that the entire race of mankind was formed by God in the loins of Adam.

Like so many theories based on preconceptions (pun intended), conjecture, and biased or otherwise misinterpreted observation, preformationist notions were awash with inconsistencies. One of those obvious even to its staunchest supporters was the implication that the lowest animal life has a divine origin, too. How could such a thing be true of contemptible creatures such as rodents, insects, and the denizens of the bottom of the seas? The answer was that animals such as ants, snails, shellfish, frogs, eels, and rats were not reproduced in this manner—they generated spontaneously from filth and corruption.

Of course, this was not a new idea. Aristotle had given it form in his contention that lower forms arise from inorganic matter and the decomposition of earth by water and heat. The theory of so-called spontaneous generation would continue to engender lively discussion and increasing debate for centuries. Even William Harvey subscribed to it. Not until Louis Pasteur provided a resounding experimental rebuttal in 1861 would its epitaph be written.

But spontaneous generation was of much less concern to the emerging scientists of that period than was human reproduction. Although the theory of preformation was very old, it had languished somewhat during the later Middle Ages and Renaissance, until Harvey inadvertently brought it back to prominence by contradicting its basic premises in his 1651 publication, *De generatione animalium* ("The Generation of Animals"). By the time the book appeared, the great experimenter was seventy years old and had suffered serious reverses, including a period of exile when Charles I, with whom he had a friend-to-friend as well as a doctor-patient relationship, was beheaded.

By the time of *De generatione animalium,* the objectivity and scientific detachment of Harvey's earlier years had begun to desert him. He was less prone to follow his own advice that researchers should "confer with our own eyes, and make our ascent from lesser things to higher" and no longer insistent that his speculations be based on hard evidence. Lapses that were rare in his earlier days (like attributing the initiation of the heartbeat to the excitement brought about by the seething forcefulness of bloodflow) were more common in his later work.

De generatione animalium started off well enough, attacking Aristotle and presenting the thesis that all life begins with the egg, a message he illustrated graphically in the volume's frontispiece, which depicts Zeus liberating a variety of tiny animals, among them a man, from an opened egg on which is inscribed the words *ex ovo omnia,* "all arises from the egg." He then went on to introduce the word *epigenesis* to describe the process of generation as he visualized it, in which some immaterial influence in the semen activates the egg into beginning its development; prior to the activation, both participants are structureless. Once this vitalistic force has acted, the process unfolds in a particular order. Epigenesis being a series of events by which the unformed matter in the egg gradually takes form—under the influence of some force in the sperm—it was a theory in which Aristotle, notwithstanding Harvey's differences with him, would surely have seen merit. But Aristotle was out of favor at the time, and Harvey was soon to join him.

The critics of epigenesis responded to Harvey with a new and improved version of the ancient preformation theory, bolstered by seemingly scientific observations. In loud voices and with bold pens, they thundered the old doctrine that the animal preexists ready-made in the male or female seed. Working with the newly popular microscope, some epigenesis advocates had already pointed out that they were seeing tissues appear as the embryo formed, those tissues then becoming enfolded into organs. Because such observations supported epigenesis, the preformationists ignored or explained them away with claims based on their own prejudgments.

Among the leading prejudgers was one of the great experimental biologists of the seventeenth century, Jan Swammerdam of Amsterdam. Swammerdam was an accomplished microscopist, who later discovered the valves in lymph ducts and was the first to describe red blood corpuscles. But like all the other notable thinkers of every era, he was a man of his time. He shared with Galen and van Helmont and even Harvey that great disability of researchers of the premodern era—the need to invoke the inscrutable. He was only fourteen when Harvey's book was published, but within less than a decade he had joined the fray.

Swammerdam sought support for the preformationist theory in Christian scripture, quoting Hebrews 7:9–10, in which Levi is said to have paid tithes when "he was yet in the loins of his father," Jacob—who had in turn preexisted in the loins of Isaac. In a 1672 publication, the thirty-five-year-old Swammerdam proclaimed his conviction that the whole race was preformed in the loins of Adam and Eve and would become extinct when the supply ran out. And this from an observer so meticulous (albeit inconsistent) that he was the first person to describe the cleavage of the fertilized ovum as the embryo begins to form. Ironically, it was Swammerdam's skill with lenses that was the major contributing factor to his being led astray. He and other preformationists of the time were lured into error by visualizing the earliest microscopic evidence of tissues and—predisposed by their interpretation of scripture—mistaking them for tiny, fully formed organs. And ironic, too, is Swammerdam's oft-quoted injunction, "We must not surmise or invent, but *discover* what nature does."

After Anton van Leeuwenhoek discovered the sperm cells, or spermatozoa, in 1674, the preformationists rushed forward to offer evidence that formed creatures were present in the newly recognized structures. Some went so far as to assert that they had *seen* tiny men within the spermatozoa. One of the researchers of the period, a naturalist named Gautier, insisted that he had observed a microscopic horse and later a rooster in the semen of those respective creatures. Perhaps such illusory observations are traceable to the altered state of mind in which the microscopists collected their semen samples, assuming that they did so after the manner of Leeuwenhoek. In a letter to the Royal Society of London, which published his observations in its *Philosophical Transactions* of November 1677, he wrote:

> What I investigate is only what, without sinfully defiling myself, remains as a residue after conjugal coitus. And if your Lordship should consider that these observations may disquiet or scandalize the learned, I earnestly beg your Lordship to regard them as private and to publish or suppress them, as your Lordship sees fit.

Earlier in the letter, Leeuwenhoek tells of having collected the specimen "immediately after ejaculation, before six beats of the pulse had intervened." Who knows what postcoital transports of afterglow may have contributed to the determined researcher's pleasured certainty in interpreting what he saw through the perhaps steamed lens of his microscope? Mrs. Leeuwenhoek, incidentally, must no doubt have been an unusually understanding woman. Either that, or she was content to be a handmaiden of science, so to speak.

Not surprisingly, the preformationists divided into two camps. The ovists believed that the individual exists preformed in the egg; the spermists (more commonly called the animalculists, because they claimed to see little fully formed animals in sperm cells) cast their vote for a spermatozoan abode.

Even when viewed with the forbearance of one who wishes not to be accused of the scholarly sin of presentism—seeing the past through eyes filled with the wonders of modern knowledge and the values of today—the arguments between the two sides seem just a bit silly. A few of the early microscopists went so far as to assert that an individual sperm contains either a male or a female animalcule, and that miniature members of the two sexes copulate with each other in the semen. The tiny offspring resulting from the union were said by these theoreticians to then develop in the womb. The evidence for such confabulations consisted of slight differences claimed to be seen near the tails of individual spermatozoa, seemingly indicating one or the other sex.

By the early eighteenth century, the preformationists had gained ascendancy over the supporters of epigenesis. In spite of some of their more extreme—or even crackpot—beliefs, the preformationists were hardly a collection of intellectual lightweights, including in their number some of the most distinguished biological investigators of the period. Men well respected both in their time and in the annals of medical history lined up as either ovists or animalculists. Among the former were researchers whose other—valid—contributions are familiar to modern students of biology and the history of science, and who are remembered for the clarity of their work.

There were fewer prominent animalculists, but some of them had towering accomplishments to their credit, including the German philosopher and mathematician Gottfried Wilhelm Leibniz and Leeuwenhoek himself. Leeuwenhoek's wrinkle on the notion of male and female sperms was to add his name to those who claimed to have identified two distinct kinds of animalcules, corresponding to the two sexes. Some said that he had discovered the homunculus of Paracelsus. Fortunately for his enduring reputation, further studies led to a change of mind, and his subsequent forceful arguments against such a possibility. One can only imagine the effect on his connubial bliss of the constantly repeated need for so many specimens—not to mention Mrs. Leeuwenhoek's patience and supply of bed linen.

But at this point, preformation doctrine dominated scientific thought, being treated as though it had arisen from the observations and experiments of the new breed of detached researchers, supported by the God-inspired interpretation of holy writ. And yet, even the most superficial analysis of its principles reveals origins that were thousands of years old. The ovists believed that the only purpose of fertilization is to supply some vital impulse that induces the fetus, already preformed in the egg, to expand. The animalculists believed that the preformed fetus is contained in the spermatozoon, with the only purpose of the ovum being to supply a proper environment for its nourishment and growth. Both groups were fond of using the analogy of a set of boxes, one inside the other inside the other, ad infinitum. (Today, we might make analogy with the Russian matryoshka dolls.) The image was not exact, but everyone knew what was meant. The obvious objection that the box analogy could only approximate truth if an individual produced but a single offspring or many that were exactly the same was ignored. Also ignored were any number of other inconsistencies, especially those that were exposed with the increasing use of the microscope after Leeuwenhoek had demonstrated what a valuable research tool it was.

The reason for such misconceptions (there it is again—it can't be avoided) is not difficult to find. The preformation doctrine was consistent with a religious philosophy that was well-nigh universally accepted at the time: The world and they that dwell therein were created in few days, along with everything required to continue in existence until the exhaustion of all that had been provided in the beginning, should the expected cataclysmic end to the world not take place. The scientists designed their theories to conform to the divine plan.

Observations were interpreted and misinterpreted in ways that were compatible with it. Thus, when the early preformation-determined microscopists began to identify little structures in the beginning stages of an embryo's development, they did not assume that these were the first evidence of tissues. In fact, they denied the possibility. Instead, they assumed the structures to be tiny human beings, in confirmation of theories long held, which conformed to the dogma of the Church. Between the misguided interpretation of observed phenomena and a certain element of arrant lying, all kinds of support were mustered for the preformation theory.

And yet, it is perhaps too harsh a judgment on these researchers to place all of the blame on them alone. The primitive magnification systems of the early microscopes lent themselves to visual aberrations resulting from the spherical shape of the lenses and their tendency to disperse daylight into the various colors of its spectrum. Magnifying the power of a lens only magnified the power of the problems. With a light source as inconsistent as the sun's rays, all sorts of objects appeared in the field of observation, some of which were not really there. To avoid such artifacts, many workers ignored microscopes entirely and used only low-power handheld lenses. In time, the evidence favoring organ development became too strong to disregard. By the mid-1700s, the preformationists were modifying their stance about preexisting persons. Gradually, they had begun to write about preexisting parts.

Amid the hodgepodge of inconsistencies in the quality of research and its interpretation during this period, a few experimental studies were nevertheless being done that even a modern-day researcher would admire for their ingenuity and value. Scientists are fond of invoking the word *elegant* to describe a particularly well-conceived and well-executed experiment, especially if it is designed with brilliant simplicity while at the same time providing definitive proof of the validity of a thesis long surmised but never quite verified. Such was the case in 1775, when the Italian physiologist Lorenzo Spallanzani demonstrated that both sperm and egg are necessary for the generation of an embryo.

Spallanzani was an ovist, convinced that the purpose of the semen is to provide some sort of immaterial stimulus to the growth of the individual already preformed in the egg. To support his beliefs, he needed some incontrovertible evidence that development cannot occur in the absence of the male contribution. That this was so had long been assumed by his fellow ovists, but no absolute proof of it had ever been produced. Though its underlying presumption of preformation was erroneous, Spallanzani, at that time a professor at the University of Pavia, carried out an inspired and direct experiment to verify the necessity of semen.

The forty-six-year-old scientist came to the problem with a long history of valid scientific accomplishment. Like so many other of the ovists, he was not a wild-eyed theorist but an experienced researcher who had made many important and correctly interpreted observations. Among the matters he had studied, first at the University of Modena and then at Pavia, were respiration, regeneration and transplantation in lower animals, gastric digestion, the functions of saliva, and the theory of spontaneous generation.

Spallanzani's ingenious plan was to dress male frogs in tiny pairs of waxed taffeta trousers and then put them together with females. The results were as he had foreseen: "The males," he wrote, "notwithstanding this encumbrance, seek the females with equal eagerness and perform, as well as they can, the act of generation; but the event is such as may be expected: the eggs are never prolific, for want of having been bedewed with semen, which sometimes may be seen inside the breeches in the form of drops."

As an encore, Spallanzani artificially fertilized the ova of frogs by placing them in direct contact with secretions squeezed out of a male's testes, a maneuver that modern-day animal rights advocates would certainly view with horror. He later repeated the experiment with tortoises, and then followed that up by impregnating a bitch with the seminal fluid of a male dog, which he injected into her uterus. By precise and even "elegant" experimentation, he had demonstrated that semen is the specific agent in fertilization, although the function of the sperm cell itself would not be understood until almost a hundred years later.

Spallanzani did all of this in the interests of supporting an underlying theory that was not only erroneous but dependent on a theological doctrine that he did not allow to enter into other areas of his work. The paradox of compartmentalization of viewpoint characterized the thinking of not only Spallanzani himself but of virtually every other experimenter who had preceded him and most of those who followed in the subsequent century. We will never be completely rid of it. Whether in the form of religious philosophy or the predisposition to interpret nature based on the personal biases and the scientific paradigm of the period, consistently pure objectivity may be a chimera. It is a goal to be strived for, but only with the realization that it is rarely attained. If it is not religion that gets in the way, it is the worldview with which one's scientific field is imbued at the time and the values placed by colleagues on interpreting observations within a generally accepted set of boundaries. And sometimes, it is an unrecognized or unacknowledged—even to oneself—personal stake in the outcome.

None of Spallanzani's fertilization studies required the aid of microscopes, so they were not subject to the optical errors that led so many researchers far afield, as it were. It would not be until the 1830s that the major optical riddles were solved by the discovery of what is called the law of aplanatic foci, enabling certain of the aberrations to be overcome. In 1826, the astronomer Giovanni Battista Amici, director of the observatory at the Royal Museum of Florence, had introduced the technique of immersing a lens in water, which made use of the principle that passing light through media of different refractory powers reduces aberration in the same way as does the human eye. In 1840, he improved the system even more, by replacing water with oil.

These changes paved the way for a remarkable era of microscopic discovery, in the course of which the basic unit of life would be shown to be the cell. Many of the hitherto-hidden truths of reproduction were also elicited in those years, gradually ending the speculations of millennia. Karl Ernst von Baer of the University of Königsberg described the mammalian ovum in 1827 and soon thereafter identified the earliest traces of the notochord, the rod-shaped length of tissue that develops into the spinal column. With enormous patience, he was able to make a long series of observations that led to his recognition, elaborated by later workers, that all tissues of the body develop from three original layers of the embryo: the inner endoderm, the middle mesoderm, and the outer ectoderm. Embryology had truly become a science.

Within a very short span of years, the entire process of fertilization, and then maturation of the embryo, had been worked out. The spermatozoon was shown to contain a nucleus and cytoplasm as had been demonstrated for the ovum some time previously. The process of the fertilized egg's segmentation into multiple cells was discovered, and finally, in 1875, a twenty-six-year-old researcher at the University of Jena in eastern Germany, Oskar Hertwig, observed the spermatozoon of a sea urchin entering the ovum. At last, the ultimate puzzle had been solved—from Hertwig's work, it was clear that fertilization occurs by a union of male and female nuclear elements. Words like *preformation, epigenesis,* and *activating spirits* were by then relegated to textbooks of the history of biology.

By the 1860s, it had become increasingly evident that the nucleus controls cell division, but the mechanism by which it does so was not understood. In 1869, it was noted that a particular chemical substance, later to be called nucleic acid, is present in the nucleus of every living cell. Its two forms, ribonucleic and deoxyribonucleic acid, were known by the 1920s. But long before that, in 1879, this nuclear substance had been given the name "chromatin," and all cell division was being called mitosis, from the Greek *mitos,* for "thread," because the chromosomes look like so many threads when seen through the microscope. It had been known since the mid-1880s that the nucleus contains the material on which heredity is based—this grew out of Hertwig's work—but it was not until 1903 that this material was theorized to be in the chromosomes. Of course, it was later shown that DNA is the genetically active part of the chromosome.

And so came to a close the thousands of years of wondering and speculation about the origin of the fetus. Of course, to call their efforts "wondering and speculation" is to ignore the certainty with which so many of the searchers put forth their formulations. The certainty was for the most part based on a combination of a strong faith in their theories' nonmaterial or religious justification and a strong faith in authority, even if it is one's own. There was a pervasive philosophy among these investigators that the proclamations of the authoritative voice were not to be contested. In corollary fashion, having become an authority one could thereafter make pronouncements without necessarily being expected to support them with what we would nowadays consider valid evidence. Although Galen was the ultimate example of this, there would be many mini-Galens to follow. When authorities disagreed, the one with the most prominent voice was likely to find far more supporters than would his adversaries.

An appreciation of the nature of real evidence and the strict criteria necessary for proof came late to the investigators of biology. The scholars who were attempting to solve the riddles presented by physics or mathematics learned much earlier than did the biologists and doctors to grapple with the necessity for critical thinking and meticulous detachment in making and interpreting observations. This was so because of the character of the problems with which they dealt and the measurability of the factors involved.

It was all very well for Francis Bacon to write in praise of inductive reasoning, or for William Harvey to advise ascending "from lesser things to higher," but the usefulness of such admonitions is limited by any observer's ability to separate wheat from chaff. Until well into the nineteenth century, researchers were feeling their way through the thicket of ignorance that obscured their path toward a disciplined analysis of the investigative problems they set for themselves. It was during these years that the scientific method was beginning to be developed. The patterns of critical thinking necessary to make real progress were anything but obvious. They were only discovered by the decades-consuming method of trial and error. But trial and error is only useful when error is recognized and a new trial is instituted. When error is obscured by religious doctrine or the booming voice of undisputed authority, it persists until religion and power relax their stranglehold enough to permit greater freedom of interpretation—to permit God and authority to oversee from more distant thrones. The more distant the god, the more dispassionate the scientist.

In a society where the constant influence of a superior and controlling divine power in all things is a given, how indeed could detachment or critical thought be brought to bear? For millennia before the spiritual focus fixed itself on one Supreme Being, it was presumed to derive from other magical or supernal sources. No matter how determined their attempts to discover the laws of nature, the men who did experiments in the seventeenth and eighteenth centuries had little doubt in their minds that God involved Himself in every phenomenon they studied.

When the unknown is thought to be unknowable, gaps in knowledge are too readily filled by fancy, so long as the fancy is consistent with faith. This crippling human predisposition, nowadays facetiously referred to as the God of the gaps syndrome, was not recognized until the latter part of the nineteenth century, and even then only by the most disciplined minds. That certain natural phenomena remain unexplained is hardly evidence that they are determined by supernatural intervention. The religious who do good science today may believe in the ultimate hand of God, but they do not invoke it to elucidate the specific physical or biological events they study or the moment-to-moment behavior of living things. Their predecessors were disinclined to question the divine source of their faith-inspired conjecturing. For too long, the questing for truth was impaired by the questing for Truth.

By the late eighteenth century, long before young people began wearing T-shirts emblazoned with the motto "Question Authority," skepticism had become a powerful force in Western culture—skepticism of the reach of God and skepticism of received wisdom. The air that real science must breathe was borne on those currents of skepticism. That new air blew away the staleness on which preformation depended; it brought in the vivifying oxygen on which progress thrives.

EPILOGUE

A single word embodies the entire foundation of Western medicine. Its three letters set the tone for a distinctive worldview of healing and for the science upon which it is based. They differentiate the structure we have come variously to call orthodox medicine, allopathic medicine, and most recently biomedicine from every other system of caring for the sick that the world has ever known. That word is *see.*

Since Western medicine's origins in ancient Greece some twenty-five hundred years ago, the perspective of its researchers and practitioners has been that the processes of both normal and diseased physiology must be *visualizable* in order to be understood in any realistic way. It is necessary, in other words, to foster a system of comprehension in which at least the mind's eye but preferably the literal eye faithfully sees the body's components as they are actually functioning. What these structures are really doing must be known—not the "idea" of what they are doing, as my Chinese colleague said of his culture's healing tradition, but what they are in fact *doing.* The Western doctor of today should be able to draw a picture of his patient's organs, tissues, and even cells, depicting the events that are happening within them. The real medicine should not truck with vague notions of immeasurable energies, inscrutable life mechanisms gone awry, or therapeutic methods so indirect that no relationship can be demonstrated between cause and effect. The aim of medicine is to describe and document every step of the process by which health becomes sickness and is then restored. The history of Western medicine has been the history of its disciples at first gradually and most recently at dizzying speed uncovering in ever more minute detail the steps within those .steps.

Some might object that the foregoing applies only to modern—nineteenth- and twentieth-century—medicine. Surely, they would say, it cannot be true of the entire panorama as far back as the historical record takes us—such notions as pneuma, coction, and the workings of humors had no basis in anything that could be seen, nor did hysteria, archei, or the sad spleen. They could not be seen because they do not exist.

Such objections are sustainable, but they can also be overruled; they are right and they are wrong. C.S. Lewis has said of writing, "I sometimes think that writing is like driving sheep down a road. If there is any gate to the left or right, the readers will most certainly go into it." The same can be said of Western medicine's long journey toward today and the future. The road is *seeing*, and the tempting gates of stray that constantly make their appearance on either side are mysticism, magical thinking, superstition, philosophy, religion, authority, rationalistic patterns of thought, preconception, misapprehension of the criteria for evidence, ambition, and—sad to tell—deceit. The gates have been slowly swinging closed since the seventeenth century, but not a single one of them has ever been completely shut, nor is such a thing likely ever to happen. Because there will be no end to medicine's journey, a few wandering members of the flock will always stray, in search of something better. And the wanderers will make all the noise they can, to encourage others to join them in the neighboring meadows.

Empedocles was the first of that very long troop who would enter upon the road of seeing, in the fifth century B.C.E. His era's philosophy and the rationalistic thinking—in which reason rather than the experience of one's senses is considered the only source of knowledge—that supported it assured that he would also be the first to slip through one of the gates, but that does not by a whit diminish either his priority or the value of his intent. His thesis that all matter is composed of various proportions of air, fire, earth, and water was not something he simply invented. It was based on a phenomenon he could see. Noting that an infinite number of hues can be created by the graduated mixing of what were in his time thought to be the four primary colors—white, black, red, and yellow—he reasoned that everything is composed of mixtures of the four "elements" that he believed to be primary.

The legendary philosopher had made an accurate observation, but faulty reasoning led him off the road and into the high grass. Like so many rationalists, he attempted to explain natural phenomena by unrestrained speculation following limited experience. His reasoning was based on the preconceptions of his time, one of which was the philosophy that a single principle unites every phenomenon of nature. To Empedocles and to tens of centuries of thinkers who followed, there was a unity between the cosmos and man—they were made of the same material and governed by the same laws. Though modern physics provides plenty of evidence to support that proposition, the early Greeks and all other civilizations went the further unjustified step of assuming that the one has suzerainty over the other—man's life is determined by events in the cosmos.

Having made an accurate, albeit small, observation about the mixing of colors, Empedocles employed his assumption of the primacy of the four so-called elements to deduce all further theory. Moreover, he was man as Claude Bernard saw man, and as so many of the innovators in this book must be seen, "Metaphysically arrogant, and thus capable of believing that the ideal creations of his mind, which express his feelings, are identical with reality." Arrogance and misused deductive reasoning of this sort would plague the thought of healers and would-be healers until the present day. Even biomedicine is not completely free of it.

What Empedocles had done was to use something he did indeed

see, to presume a structure he had no way of confirming. This rationalistic form of logic would, in fact, remain the prevalent mode of medical theory making until empiricism—dependence only on reproducible observation and experience—overtook it relatively recently. The heritage of rationalism remains.

Rationalists theorize entire systems of explanation. Empiricists, on the other hand, restrict themselves to what is seen and limit their few speculations to those supported by their own sightings or those of similar-minded observers. They are content to proceed in short steps, inducing truth from the progressive accumulation of facts. In his well-named *Cogitata et visa* ("Things Thought of and Things Seen") of 1607, Francis Bacon wrote, "Empiricists are like ants, they collect and put to use; but rationalists, like spiders, spin threads out of themselves." It is the "out of themselves" that constitutes the operative thought. Having made his observation, Empedocles felt justified in using his innate reasoning powers to spin the threads of an entire webwork of theory. The leap in his reasoning was supported by contemporary convention; this is the way things were done in the fifth century B.C.E. Like every other of the innovators described in this book, Empedocles was a person of his time, a time of philosophy and rationalism. A man can no more shed his skin than shed the mode of thinking of the era in which he lives.

Still, regardless of his understandable errors, Empedocles did proceed from an observation that he and everyone else could confirm. The result of mixing paints could be *seen*. He had led the way to the right road. Contrast this with the historic origins of such theoretical formulations as chi, homeopathy, and reflexology, to cite only a few examples. These are concepts whose biologic mechanisms are confirmable neither by a preceding observation that stands the test of experiment nor by any evidence that has ever been seen by the eye or measured by the mind.

The humors, too, were visible fluids. It took a bit of a stretch to account for black bile, but once that stretch was made, the reasonableness of the theory of humors was thereafter unquestioned. The black stools of slow intestinal bleeding, the coffee-ground vomit of certain gastric disturbances, the foul black discharge of an advanced and ulcerated rectal, breast, cervical, or skin cancer—all of these qualified. Moreover, they were apt to be accompanied by melancholy—*melas chole,* black bile.

The greatest of the early see-ers came center stage shortly after Empedocles's death in 430 B.C.E. These were the apostles of the Hippocratic system, who made meticulous observations of the visible signs and symptoms of their patients' diseases. They based their diagnoses only on what they could see. Empedocles had formulated theories based on his conception that all observable phenomena have natural causes, eschewing any explanation derived from either religion or superstition. The Hippocratics followed him in their rejection of supernature. Not for them such influences as sin, ghostly spirits in disarray, or the wrath of the gods. They studied the observable effects of such factors as food, climate, and state of mind. The Hippocratic physician took note of hot skin, fast pulse, dry tongue, yellow stool, foul-smelling urine, and a jaundiced eye. Though their acceptance of humoral explanations kept them almost as much in thrall to philosophy and rationalism as was Empedocles, they knew what clinical evidence to look for at the bedside and they could describe it for their students and posterity. Their aim was to replace the mythology of health and disease with truth, as they could learn it by painstaking observation of nature. Because they relied only on the objectivity of what could be seen, they became skilled at predicting the course of a disease and the likely outcome of its treatment. Prognostication became one of their most highly prized skills. Such an ability was impossible for those without eyes to see.

Though much of Galen's theorizing was the product of empiricism gone adrift into philosophy and authoritarian arrogance, he too at least attempted to base his medicine on what he could see. He publicly repeated his various animal experiments over and over, always reproducing the same results in a manner—as he boastfully proclaimed—that could be emulated by anyone who had the skill to do the dissections. He was led astray by the rationalistic thinking of his period, by his notions of religion, by driving ambition, and certainly by the imperiousness of his asserted authority. And yet, the one consistency running through his thought was its origin in reproducible observations.

So dominant was Galen's authority that real progress stopped for fifteen centuries, until Vesalius published *De fabrica*. That book was the very incarnation of seeing. By meticulous observation at one after another cadaver dissection and the commissioning of skillful drawings of all that he demonstrated, Vesalius in 1543 bade his fellow physicians to once again take up the obligation of seeing. They must believe nothing, he proclaimed, that they could not bring before their own eyes. The example of Vesalius was a major stimulus to the great advances in science that would occur in the seventeenth century. Of these, two were most notable for medicine. The first was William Harvey's discovery of the circulation, growing entirely out of what he could see and what he could measure. The second was the empiricist admonition of Francis Bacon that the elucidation of natural phenomena requires the study of facts via the gradual ascent inherent in inductive thought, which would come to mean a process of observation, hypothesis, and experiment—and only then theory. From this grew the concept commonly known as the scientific method. The book in which he presented his approach was appropriately entitled *Novum organum* ("The New Instrument").

There is no need to burden this text with the further travelogue of the Western physician's eventful journey along the road of seeing, which in time acquired the assistance of advances in chemistry, physics, and technology. These would make it possible to visualize smaller and smaller bits of the structure that is a human being. Those minutenesses not capable of being observed directly were understood by means of their effects and manifestations, in laboratory studies that brought all to visibility. When today's biomedical physician describes a process inside the body, he attempts to detail every event that is actually taking place within the organs involved and the cells of which they are composed. Even the interactions among molecules often fall within the field of his indirect scrutiny. One way or another, his goal is to see everything.

But it is obvious from a reading of this book that medicine's journey, even during and after the so-called scientific revolution of the seventeenth century, never did become a steady progression that swept all healers and researchers along with it. Though fewer in number and lesser in consequence, driftings through those open gates continued. Vagrants found their way to error. Concessions to mysticism, illogic, and imagination did not end. The van Helmonts, the Glissons, and the Swammerdams had plenty of company as they roamed the fields and forests off the road of seeing. Very few of them ever realized that they were lost.

There is one overriding factor which more than any other led to the peregrinations into the thickets of mistaken theories: the continuing search for a single unifying explanation of the behavior of all life and matter. We seek it still, though many of us are convinced that it has been found. The faithful find it in God, and the reductionist physicists have recently become convinced that it is to be understood in terms of fundamental forces and elementary particles.

Before tracing the evolution of humankind's strivings to discover the ultimate unity, it might be good to describe the currency in which today's physicists deal. Their conceptions of atoms and the cosmos can perhaps serve as a mirror in which to reflect backward on the millennia of searching—searching for the fundamental principles that science now appears to be bringing to light.

And now for the argot of modern physics. Some of the scientific language that follows, and certainly the underlying general outline, will seem familiar to everyone who has come this far in the narrative. The language and the outline of modern physics are reminiscent of previous all-encompassing theories men have made in their never-ending pursuit of some single overarching truth that explains all. There are two possible lessons in this similarity, and they contradict each other. Either the intuitive reach of man's mind is so profound that it has always sensed the unity of all matter and energy that is now being demonstrated by the physicists; or the unity now being so scientifically elucidated is a chimera, and just another of the inescapable consequences of a fantasized image of the universe that is somehow programmed into our species—a perception that may be genetically imposed, culturally transmitted, or a combination of both. In other words, perhaps the unity exists only in the scientific imagination, as a result of interpreting data to fit a preconceived idea, a matter more of perception than of reality. Though there is every reason to believe that the first lesson is the correct one, we ignore the second at our peril, no matter its seeming improbability.

Read on, and think of Empedocles. Read on, and keep in mind that no one has ever actually seen any of the structures or energies about to be described. Their existence, though predicated on the soundest of mathematical and physical principles and supported by their usefulness in experimental settings—is nevertheless still theoretical.

Herewith the testimony of the physicists: The evidence of modern science is that everything and everyone is made up of combinations of three families of elementary particles and four fundamental forces that hold them together. The forces are gravity, electromagnetism (the source of light and other radiation), and the so-called strong and weak forces (which determine the structure of the atomic nucleus). From the behavior of forces and particles, today's scientists are convinced that the time is rapidly approaching when they can present what they like to think of as a single "theory of everything," which they call the GUT, for grand unified theory. Think again of Empedocles.

In this formulation, the only difference between an earthworm and the wall you see when you look up from this book—or between you and that star twinkling in the night sky—is the way in which the forces and particles are organized and interact. It is a notion that would have done Empedocles proud. Of course, there are huge numbers of additional details and still plenty of disagreements within this very general presentation of the unity of all things, but the followers of Empedocles also spoke of details, and there were certainly plenty of schools of thought into which they were divided. Both the ancient Greeks and the modern scientists have approached their theories with the equivalent underlying assurance, that the entire universe is all made of the same stuff, governed by the same rules. It is the search for the components of the sameness that has brought philosophical and scientific thinkers of every stripe and every era into the same camp.

But there is one enormous and crucial difference between the respective processes by which scientists of today and the earliest of thinkers have reached their conclusions. To a modern researcher, there is no final answer and certainly no final cause, only a final theory. The final theory is determined at the end—the finale, if you will—of a long series of ascensions from lesser to greater, in the gathering of facts. It is, in other words, the result of induction. Empedocles and the men of his time began their cogitations in exactly the opposite way. First, the grand theories were created, and by some the grand causes. The details which led from them were filled in later. The final theory or cause initiated, rather than concluded, the process. It was the fount from which the thinkers deduced, interpreting every observation in its light and in turn using those observations to support the validity of the final concept.

A second difference between the ancient and modern processes is the capacity of the final theory to evolve, once it is discovered by induction. When the final theory or cause comes first, on the other hand, the system is immutable. For a scientist, final is never Final. In fact, modification and even change of lesser or greater degree is inevitable as new observations are made and new ways of interpreting them appear. The theoretics of an Empedocles or of a van Helmont, on the other hand, sprang fully formed from the forehead of their creator, like Minerva from Jupiter, and they did not change with the years. Like all systems of nonorthodox medicine, they were forever fixed.

But these were matters not well understood until the past few centuries. In very earliest—what we often call primitive—times, there were no tools, either physical or intellectual, by the use of which man might understand his surroundings. Sense had to be made of the vast number of phenomena encountered every hour of an often perilous existence. And if sense could not be made, man at least needed ways to deal with the capriciousness of the stimuli that assailed his perceptions and of events over which he had so little control. Explanations had to be found that could be comprehended by everyone. They took the form of sprites, demons, ghosts, and the gods of places and things. These were erratic, often unfriendly, and given to playing tricks and inflicting misfortunes if not propitiated with sacrifices, incantations, and amulets. Among the misfortunes was disease. Superstitions arose, through which man thought he had found answers and ways to deal with the mysteries of his world. If disease was caused by magical forces, then magic must be used in their cure. Magic and medicine were intertwined, and that intertwining is with us still.

Earliest man looked around him and saw things move. He himself moved. Things inside his body moved. Even the moon and the stars moved. But he recognized that there were different kinds of motion. The motion of animals and the waters came from within themselves. The heavenly bodies and the branches of trees seemed to be propelled by something external. If living things moved on their own, they must contain an animating force; the movement of the waters would appear to be caused by something similar. The concept that would later come to be called anima, or psyche, thus came into being, and before long was elaborated by increasingly sophisticated thinkers into spirit, an essence that not only animated but gave life and was part of the ultimate source of all matter and energy, a divine afflatus associated with the cosmos and the configurations of the heavenly bodies. *Psyche,* the Greek word for "soul" or "spirit," is derived in fact from an Indo-European root indicative of breathing. From his first breath of existence, man had inhaled an effluvium of that supernal atmosphere of the cosmos, and he came to call it pneuma, the vital breath. And thus was born religion, but superstition was its older brother. Some would say that superstition was its father.

And then, there emerged the concept that everything in the universe has a single all-encompassing explanation. From that point forward, all was interpreted to have a purpose, because the decrees of a great artisan or demiurge had created and maintained the world. But still, the purpose of believing in a purpose was to mitigate the fear of the unknown, the incomprehensible, and the unpredictable that had stalked man's steps since the beginning. The metaphysical continued to be invoked to explain the physical, because there was no other way. When the belief in purpose was added, faith took on form and structure. A theology began to develop. Religion headed down a separate pathway from superstition, but the older brother's—or father's—influence refused to disappear.

In time, great thinkers—of whom Empedocles was the most prominent—entered the arena and began to look at the phenomena of nature in a novel way. Whatever may be the authority of a divine power, they proposed, man should seek the explanations for nature within nature itself. Perhaps the demiurge had ordained the world and left it to run on its own, having created it of the matter and the energy that is part of the eternal cosmos. If this is so, there must be natural laws, and they are discoverable. Even if they were promulgated by a god, he too obeys them.

The human body came to be seen as an instrument of the soul, and the soul an expression of divine will and relationship with the entire universe. In every sense, therefore, the human body was identified with the cosmos and interpreted as its reflection and even a part of it—a microcosm of the macrocosm, and both were incorporated into the same living thing, the thing given life and meaning by its soul. To the religious, this was confirmation of God; to the Greek forebears of scientific thinking, it was that, too, but it also signified a universal physics of nature; to the philosophers who were the earliest of those forebears, even the soul was part of the unity—the most important part.

And thus began the first glimmerings of science. Man in the classical period and Middle Ages attempted to build a philosophical structure of material things, while proclaiming the certainty that his spiritual essence made him unique—made him different from all that surrounded him. That spiritual essence also put him at one with the universe, because its ultimate source was the supernal and the cosmos. He called on it and the god it confirmed, whenever he came up against phenomena he could not yet explain by his new investigations. After the late Renaissance, the number of those unknowable phenomena became progressively smaller, as man uncovered ever more of nature's secrets, and needed less of God to help him understand. Faith found an arena of its own, created from the moral precepts, the theological philosophies, and the formalized structure that had begun to grow at the time of its beginnings. In certain ways it became stronger, and more independent of being justified by the residual ignorance of nature's ways. The gaps that men filled with theories of supernatural things became smaller.

But the temptation to explain nature on the basis of the metaphysical remained great. Even the most perceptive of educated people— and some scientists too—continued to succumb to it until well into the nineteenth century, as we have again and again noted in this narrative of seeing gone wrong. But after the publication in 1859 of Darwin's *Origin of Species,* the split became virtually complete. No longer could any scientist expect to be taken seriously should he invoke supernature in his theories. Religion and science not only parted ways completely but began a campaign of hostilities against each other that is sometimes so acrimonious as to diminish its participants.

Neither side need bother. Those who see religion and science as being mutually contradictory would do well to remember the observation made by F. Scott Fitzgerald in an entirely different context in his essay "The Crack-Up." He wrote, "[T]he test of a first-rate intelligence is the ability to hold two opposed ideas in the mind at the same time, and still retain the ability to function." Indeed, the world of science does not lack for devout believers in God, and there have been prominent scientific thinkers among the clergy. But Fitzgerald's is only a first approach to reconciliation, and an incomplete one at that. Of far greater value is the recognition that these two systems of thought are independent of each other, and for that reason without grounds for conflict. They are not, in fact, opposed. They require mental processes and assumptions that are neither congruent nor even parallel. The observable, provable, repeatable, and measurable have nothing to do with the unknowable, ineffable, mystical, and inexpressible. Their respective truths cannot be judged by the same criteria. Though either side may have reason to reject some or all of the other's formulations, there are plenty of thoughtful minds at ease with themselves that consider the two systems to be complementary rather than antagonistic.

It has been my observation that the antagonism between the two is more likely to come from the scientists and like-minded people than from the religious. And I wonder about that. What is so irksome about another person's faith? Is the intolerance a kind of intellectual arrogance directed at minds perceived to be simpler or at least less sophisticated than one's own? It ill behooves a man or woman self-placed on a higher intellectual plane to descend to combat with those he or she deems less qualified or cerebrally gifted. That fact alone should still much of the hauteur, even if the cynical mumblings among colleagues continue to be heard in the lab or the academic hallway. Why is it not below the supposed dignity of the lofty rational mind to be concerned with overcoming the ignorance of the scientifically unwashed? What is the real basis for the attacks?

Although imperious disdain may be a factor, I believe there is a much more fundamental reason that so many confirmed believers in science should be so outspoken in their denigration of religious precepts. The trained mind of a person committed to scientific thought perhaps realizes better than most—even if the realization is not on a conscious level—that its detachment and objectivity, not to say the foundation of its analytical powers, are not characteristics that have come without difficulty. It realizes that logical thought is easily sidetracked, and requires eternal vigilance to maintain. It realizes further that any concessions made to so much as a taste of mysticism have the potential to begin a process by which the carefully constructed edifice of the scientific approach is endangered. It realizes still further that we are closer to magical thinking than most of us know. No one is immune. In times of threat, sickness, need, or desire, even those of us most imbued with reason fall all too easily into the patterns of magical musings and sometimes even retreat into superstition. With the least of provocations, we may abandon the logical thinking it took so many centuries for humankind to acquire. This is quite a different thing from turning to religious faith for solace or strength or to clarify one's thought. But skeptical scientists do not see the difference. To them, magical thinking is inherent in religion, and therefore religion is a clear and ever-present danger. They fight it because they fear it, not only in others but in themselves. They know that the recourse to magic lurks within. With the siren's tempting wiles wafts a contaminant that can spoil the purest intent. For such reasons, the reasonable mind sometimes becomes unreasonable in the face of faith.

And what about the religious? Why do they attempt logic and reason to prove matters which by their very nature are beyond any logic and higher than all reason? Why do so many of them feel that it is beholden on them to apply the rules of proof and evidence in arguments for which such rules were never intended? Is not faith enough? If the experience of religion is as personal as it is said to be, it matters not a whit that skeptics do not accept its basic structure of supernatural authority, on the grounds that it has no evidence to support it. Is that not why we use the word *faith*?

And finally, one must deal with the obverse of the scientist's concerns about religion, which consists of the threat that some of the faithful feel when confronted by the findings of science. To respond to this, I call on a descendant of a long line of New England ministers, whose resignation from the pulpit at the age of thirty-five did not at all lessen his devotion to God. Withal, he was an avid exponent of science. On March 4, 1831, Ralph Waldo Emerson, then the pastor of Boston's Second Church, wrote in his journal, "The Religion that is afraid of science dishonours God and commits suicide." One might say with equal fervor that the science that is afraid of religion dishonors its claim to detachment and sows the seed of its own destruction.

The foregoing paragraphs have been a tangent, but a necessary one. Throughout this book, one after another example has appeared of the ways in which supernatural beliefs have clouded the eyes of science and diverted it through a gateway of error. Whether instigated by magic, superstition, or misapplied religion, the underlying reason for every one of the misadventures has been the same. In each case, a mystical cause has been invoked when there is no other ready explanation for some observed phenomenon. When something is not understood, it has been easiest to see the hand of God on it.

The tradition of fanciful and magical formulations lives on, and it should not. What I have earlier called the god of the gaps has no place in modern thought. One is not justified in defending religious belief by pointing to the remaining mysteries of nature, even should the furthest reach of man's mind at present see no possibility of their solution. The history of science has been the history of elucidating phenomena that in their time seemed beyond human comprehension, and there is no reason to think that the seemingly more complex mysteries of today will not similarly fall before the continuing onslaught of scientific curiosity. There is a worldview of difference between a final theory and a Final Cause.

Religion and science should stay out of each other's bailiwicks. What is needed is not a debate between them but a conversation. Perhaps out of it could come a clarification of what is true religious thought and what are the residual impedimenta of superstition and magical thinking. Religion might be cleansed by such an ongoing conversation, and science made to understand that faith is not its enemy.

And perhaps, too, the character of mankind's thought might come to be addressed. Why, after all these millennia, do we still so easily turn to magical ideation when faced with uncertainty or lack of knowledge? We should recognize and accept that critical thinking and logical analysis are alien to our nature. They must be taught, and they must be constantly reinforced. If there is no other lesson in this book, this is the one that should be remembered. Humankind came late to reason, and even later to scientific logic. We are still their reluctant partner. It is because of their knowledge of the ease with which primitive instincts escape from repression that so many scientists mistakenly attack religious faith.

Superstition and religion began their journey together and have never completely separated. Magic and medicine have done the same. In this I include Western medicine, but above all else I refer to those other varieties of healing that have always captured the human imagination. Living fossil forms are everywhere around us, of every unconfirmable method that has ever been used in the treatment of illness— and many that are modern in their claims but ancient in their appeal to the irrational currents that so effortlessly surface in our thinking. We are beset nowadays with a host of nonstandard techniques of healing, ranging from pure quackery to forms of traditional medicine from which nuggets of real value might be extracted were they only subjected to the same scrutiny as biomedicine. The very fact that so many of today's nonorthodox practices are without proof of their validity or their basic assumptions makes them more attractive to many of their adherents. That their purported mechanisms of action require a leap of fantasy is at the heart of their survival. Enshrouded in the mystery we humans find so appealing, they live on in various forms, generation after generation.

Whether in the Greek insistence on purgings, the Paracelsian doctrine of similars, or the undifferentiated herbalism that has existed in all ages, the roots of today's unorthodox healing methods run deep. Strains of the old refrains are heard everywhere, and they are familiar to anyone who will but take the trouble to listen. Some of them have well-known names and require training to practice, like homeopathy, chiropractic, and much that comes under the heading of traditional medicine. Others are easily mastered, and their unskilled avatars dispense advice and nostrums without benefit of any but the most superficial knowledge. When they succeed, it is usually because recovery was assured even without them—the vast majority of sickness does, after all, get better by itself. The Greeks knew this. In the Hippocratic text *Epidemics* we find this: "Nature, without instruction or knowledge, does what is necessary." The very word *physician* is derived from the Greek *physis,* meaning "nature," and in this oft-neglected fact is the core of healing's secret.

In other cases, the dispensers of the alternative do achieve results that might not have otherwise occurred, and that has to do with the practitioner's authority and the patient's belief system. In either case, the ancient fallacy of reasoning known as *post hoc ergo propter hoc* takes hold, and what is subsequent is deemed to be consequent. Since our species first tried to heal, we have uncritically attributed recoveries to our efforts and anointed as though they were proven the methods used. Anecdote is more powerful than data, and will always be. When we slip from logical thinking, we believe what we need—or wish—to believe.

Anecdote achieves its power because so much of it is testimony. The untrained listener cannot resist the appeal of testimony, laden as it is with emotion and the conviction of the healed. We hear it every day. The most detached of us find difficulty in turning our thoughts from it, and back to critical evaluation and reliable statistical methods. Like *post hoc* reasoning, testimony has ever stood as a foundation stone of error.

We study the fallacies of reasoning of our medical forebears, fallacies they fell into despite their determination to *see* the structures and processes they were trying to explain. With the wisdom of present knowledge, we try to resist the impulse to criticize them for not recognizing what is obvious today. Though we acknowledge that they were creatures of their various times and therefore subject to mysticism, authority, undeveloped analytical methods—not to mention a poverty of technology—and the entire constricting box called preconception, we nevertheless on some level have reservations about their inability to have risen above such influences. The mere fact of recognizing the impossibility of overcoming the worldview of one's era does not stop us from a vague intolerance of their misconceptions, though we know that we have no right.

Historians call this sort of thinking "presentism"—judging the past by the standards of the present. It is not the tendency to presentism, however, that should give us pause in feeling superior to the past, but rather failure to recognize the fact that even biomedicine carries with it the heritage of magic. Paradoxically, in view of all that I have been saying here, that may not be such a bad thing.

The spokesmen for Western medicine articulate a vision of their art in which it is barely an art at all, but has almost totally become a science. To anyone who has spent the days of a long career at the bedsides of the sick, that conceit is ludicrous, and in any event does not describe a situation to be desired. The magic that has always been intertwined with medicine is no less a part of healing today than it has ever been—it simply comes in a different costume. To take the obvious illustration, the red body paint and extravagant headdress of the primitive healer have been replaced with the white coat, and the rattles and rods with a stethoscope. Whatever the clinical value of the modern doctor's electronic space-age armamentarium, its unspoken other usefulness lies in symbolism, the symbolism of authority.

Authority has always lain at the foundation of healing. The modern hospital, now frequently with the trappings of an academic medical center, is a magical place. It contains the aura of the ancient Aesculapian temple of healing. The white-coated or scrub-suited physician, remote in his clinical distance and austere in the mysteries of the arcana he controls, is the equivalent of the temple priest. What is more enshrouded in the mystery we humans crave than the complex impedimenta of diagnosis and treatment to which today's physician alone has access? The fact that he is nowadays often a she has hardly detracted from the atmosphere of specialized and esoteric knowledge upon which she can call. Incantations are heard, in a privileged language that only the priests and their retainers are able to speak. The colored pills of two centuries ago are still colored, and their recondite names are as redolent of the occult as ever, even if now chemical rather than botanical. Cure, which in the Aesculapian temple was revealed in a dream, still often occurs during sleep, a sleep induced by means of potions administered at the direction of the healer. The patient lies still as though dead, his life-sustaining pneuma having been replaced by pungent gases wafted directly into his chest, the seat of the soul that has abandoned him in his sickness. During unconsciousness, his skin is ritually scarified and the restless internal organs are soothed. When the cure has been effected, he awakens and is revived by the vital breath taken in from the cosmos, which restores the spirit lost in the process of sickness.

Such analogies are, of course, exaggerated—but only a little. Biomedicine is wrapped in a hand-me-down cloak that is as old as civilization, and much of its fabric serves the unknowing need for mystery that seems to be an inherent characteristic of our species. This is as it has always been and as it will always be. Even today, magic is often part of the cure, and in some situations it is the entire cure. Those of us so quick to criticize the foundations of non-Western medicine should recognize that we employ some of its tricks—unwittingly perhaps—in our own sanctums of healing. If we understood this better, we might make more effective use of them, or at least be less cha-grined that medicine will never be totally scientific. There is, of course, a vast difference between utilizing magic deliberately as an ad-junct to science and its use by those who rely on it to *replace* science and make claims for it which cannot be substantiated by the rigid stan-dards that should be applied to such matters.

Galen said it for the ages: "He cures most successfully in whom the people have the most confidence." Every doctor has been witness to this phenomenon, unexplainable though it may yet be. Such cures are related to the notion of expectation: it is well known and has been clinically documented that the patient who expects to get better is more likely to do so than the patient in the next bed who expects to get worse. Whatever other factors determine expectation, confidence in one's physician is surely a major ingredient, if not *the* major ingre-dient.

Expectation is a kind of authority—it authorizes the patient to re-cover, and much of it originates in the authority of the physician to provide that authorization. This is the basis of the so-called placebo ef-fect, as old as the art of healing and as magical as the expulsion of an excess of yellow bile by powerful purges—or in another culture, the overwrought dance of a pigment-smeared shaman. The word itself—*placebo*—is Latin for "I will please," and refers to any inactive medica-tion or procedure administered only to gratify a patient's desire for treatment. It is given to "please" the patient. The doctor may know that the therapy is scientifically worthless, or its lack of efficacy may be realized only later. Whatever beneficial effect it has (which in a variety of types of modern studies has ranged from 21 percent to a remark-able 58 percent, depending on the disease, the placebo, and the way the study is done) is due to suggestion—the suggestion of the author-ity from whom it comes.

But another meaning of placebo should be considered, and it has to do with the way in which a patient pleases his doctor by getting well. We have the Hippocratic writings to thank for this interpretation: "Some patients, though conscious that their condition is perilous, re-cover their health simply through their contentment with the goodness of the physician." One of the most quoted studies of the placebo effect is W. R. Houston's classic 1938 paper, published in the *Annals of Internal Medicine* a year after he presented it before the membership of the American College of Physicians. Its very title illustrates the physician's role in his patient's recovery: "The Doctor Himself as a Therapeutic Agent." Houston reiterated for his audience something that most of them already knew, namely that "the great lesson, then, of medical history is that the placebo has always been the norm of medical practice," until the modern era. All but a few of those herbal concoctions, pukings, bleedings, doses of mercury, sulfur, or hellebore root were for naught, except as they turned on something in a patient's brain that actuated—and was actuated by—his will to recover. They were, in fact, placebos. In other words, until recently the doctor was a magician.

He is one still. The difference between then and now is that today we know enough science so that Western physicians should be able to apply modern versions of the ancient placebo phenomenon selectively and therefore much more effectively. Though we may giggle and scoff at our centuries of predecessors, they have much to teach us. Led through the gates of error by philosophy, rationalism, superstition, and religion though they were, the doctors of yesteryear nevertheless left an inadvertent and unappreciated heritage. As Houston put it, in a brief burst of poetic parallelism, "[T]heir learning was a learning in how to deal with men. Their skill was a skill in dealing with the emotions of men." This is what the homeopaths and reflexologists and chiropractors, too, have to teach us, for it is the only real thing they can offer, in spite of their protestations of scientific validity. The magic and the mystery that biomedicine thinks it has discarded are with us yet. We need to look up and see that truth, so that our patients—and we too—can benefit from it.

This book has been a catalog of the intrusion of the spiritual into the temporal. In earliest times, the two were inseparable, but with the Greeks came the realization that the phenomena of nature might best be studied independent of celestial explanation. They were mistaken in their certainty that the influence of the supernatural could long be kept out of their medical philosophy. It never really left, and in a few hundred years it was back in full flower, with Galen writing of a god who made man, and seeing His purpose in the structure of every organ. When the rudiments of science appeared, they arose through a nimbus of religious thought and metaphysics. Long beyond the point when men knew that the respective spheres of faith and science should leave hold of each other, the vaporous mists of religious influence—and persistent superstition, too—continued to cloud the thinking of those who would probe nature's secrets. The influence was baleful, but neither permanent nor lethal. By the beginning of the nineteenth century, it was largely a thing of the past, but its interferences left a heritage of mistrust, particularly after Darwin. Even the most devout scientist of today leaves his faith at the door when he enters the laboratory each morning, and puts it back on along with his coat when the day's work is done. And that is as it should be.

Religion does not belong in the laboratory, but it should have an honored place at the bedside. More than 90 percent of Americans believe in God, and that number surely rises when major sickness strikes. The familiar strains of religion can, as Houston so eloquently told his assembled colleagues, "express in fit and beautiful words many truths that seem to fade and perish when put into the clumsy terms of science." It is not for a physician to question a patient's faith, but to support it. A skeptic myself, I have seen the wonders that faith can bring to the desperately ill and to their families. Even when it does not lessen the pain or fear of death, it comforts—and consoles both the living and the dying for what is being lost. And strange to say, it somehow comforts the hardened physician, too, to see that the human mind is capable of such sublime belief.

Earlier, the word *physician* was traced to the Greek *physis*, meaning "nature." But the ancients left us with more than just that, and it must be considered. All of what pertained to nature they called *physikos*, and from this is derived the name of the modern discipline that studies the physical laws of the universe—physics. Physicians and physics are thus seen to be connected. And so, in going back to the Greeks and their theory of the unity of all things, linguistic derivation illuminates the road leading from then to now, just as the ancient thesis is revealed to be at one with the discoveries of turn-of-the-twenty-first-century science. By this I mean that the etymological relationship between physician and physics can be seen as a metaphor: the human body that must be healed is once again shown to be united with the immensity of the cosmos of which it is a part.

We are traveling on the same road—first of superstition, and after Empedocles ever more of seeing—that we have been on since our forebears were first disquieted by the animals they thought were moving about inside them. That road, which has taken us from primitive fears to modern physics, signifies our continuity with everything that has gone before. It reminds us that whether we believe ourselves to be children of God or children of nature, our past is bound up with our future, and we are bound up with one another.

INDEX

Christianity compared with theories
of, 210
on coction and chyle, 57, 59, 72, 199
Descartes and, 75
on fertilization, 236–38
on heart, 199–201, 204–5
on humors, 51, 58, 146, 149–50,
209
on hysteria, 221–22
influence of, 57–59, 117, 120, 123,
198–99, 208–9, 251
life of, 57–58
on liver, 57, 95, 112, 116–17, 133,
147, 199–200
on lungs, 199–200
Paracelsus on, 125, 126, 128
on speech, 199
on spleen, 145, 147–48, 150–51, 154,
161
on uterus, 216, 225
galenicals, 117
gallbladder, 116, 131
used in divination, 113
galvanometer, 205
gas, van Helmont's theory of, 66, 69,
234*n*
gaster, 39
gastric wall, 39, 79
gastrointestinal imaging, 81
Gelfoam, 97
"Generation of Animals, The"
(Harvey), 242–43
Genesis, Book of, 73, 240
genital massage, as treatment for hysteria, 222–23, 225–26
genitals, 211–12
votive images of, 229–30
Gilgamesh epic, 110
GI series, 81
Glisson, Francis, 130–31, 259
Glisson's capsule, 102–3, 131
globus hystericus, 216
glucose, 133
glycogen, 133
grand unified theory (GUT), 260–61
gravity, 260
Greeks, ancient:
Alexandrian school and, 196–98,
215–16, 233, 237
dissection by, 54, 55
on emotions in disease, 152
on fertilization, 233–34
on heart, 192

on humors, *see* humors
influences on, 48, 49
microcosm/macrocosm thesis and,
114
mysticism of, 48–50
philosophical systems of, 19, 53,
65–66
Prometheus myth of, 111
spleen as viewed by, 47, 142–43,
145–46
on uterus, 212–16
votive objects of, 229–30
see also specific individuals
Green, Matthew, 155
Gregory the Great, 240
GUT (grand unified theory), 260–61

Haggith, 143
Halevi, Judah, 153
Harvey, William, 116, 130, 144, 154,
163, 189, 194, 201–4, 209, 224, 251,
258
on epigenesis, 242–43
scientific importance of, 201, 203,
206
heart, 163–206
Aristotle on, 61, 116, 193
Alexandrians on, 197–98
ancient Greeks on, 192
arrhythmia in, 176–80
atrium of, 169, 176–81, 205, 209
emotions as arising from, 195–96
in experiments on dogs, 165–68
Galen on, 199–201, 204–5
head vs., 193–94
in metaphor, 191–92
mitral stenosis and, 169–70
mitral valvulotomy and, 168–82
myogenic theory of, 204–5
prehistoric awareness of, 183–84
as seat of love, 195–96
solidity of, 192–93
as source of blood, 51
as source of semen, 234
sympathy between stomach and,
61–62
ventricles of, 169, 177, 200, 205
heartbeat, 163–64, 184, 192, 201,
204–5, 209
"heartburn," origin of, 61
Hebrews, Book of, 243
hemostats, 92, 94, 101, 107
Henri de Mondeville, 62

Henry II, King of France, 219
hepatic artery, 95–97, 107
hepatoscopy, 112–14
Heracles, Prometheus myth and,
    111
herbal remedies, for liver, 117–19
Herbert, George, 118–19
Herophilus, 55, 237
Hertwig, Oskar, 250
Hippocrates, 120, 149
    death of, 55, 146
    Egyptian influence on, 48
    on fertilization, 235, 236
    Paracelsus on, 125, 126
    Sydenham as follower of, 224
Hippocratics, 49, 50, 53, 118, 193, 199,
    208–9
    on hysteria, 220–21
    on placebo effect, 271–72
    on prolapsed uterus, 228
    in rejection of supernatural, 257
    on spleen, 145–46
homeopathy, 124, 127, 256
homeostasis, 50
Homer, 183–84, 192
homunculus, 238, 246
honey, 187
horseback riding, 225
Houston, W. R., 272
humors, 48–54, 114, 145–46, 149–51,
    154, 187, 207–8, 256–57
    described, 51–52
    disease ascribed to imbalance in,
        52–54, 186
    Galen on, 51, 58, 146, 149–50, 209
    seasonal effects on, 53, 150
    uterus and, 214
    words derived from, 52
Hunter, John, 78
    on iatrophysicists vs. iatrochemists,
        76
    on living principle, 77
Hygeia, 48
hypertrophy, 40
hypochondria:
    hysteria and, 217, 224
    as symptom of Spleen, 155, 158
hystera, 212, 213, 219
hysteria, 214–28
    ancient Egyptians on, 220–21
    Aretaeus on, 214–15, 217
    Buchan on, 217–19
    as "contagious," 218–19

female semen as cause of, 221–23,
    225
Freud on, 219, 226
Galen on, 221–22
genital massage as treatment for,
    222–23, 225–26
Hippocratics on, 220–21
hypochondria and, 217, 224
in men, 219, 226
in Middle Ages, 218, 222
modern abandonment of term,
    226–27
Paré's treatments for, 222–23
psychosexual explanations of, 220–26
psychotherapy for, 219, 226–27
sexual intercourse as treatment for,
    220, 221–22, 223
St. Vitus' dance and, 223–24
Sydenham on, 224–25
"Hysteria: A Clinical Guide to
    Diagnosis" *(Ciba Clinical Symposia),*
    227
hystericohypochondriacum, 217

iatrochemistry:
    alchemy and, 75, 120–21, 123–24
    iatrophysics vs., 74–77
    van Helmont as founder of, 65,
        74–75, 120, 127
iatrophysics, 74–77
    Baglivi as proponent of, 75–77
iatros, 65
Idomeneus, 184
Iliad (Homer), 184, 192
incubi, 218
India, Vedic texts of, 121
inflammation, diagnosis of, 31
Innocent VIII, Pope, 218
Institute for Experimental Medicine at
    St. Petersburg, 81
insulin, 133
internal lavage, 188
intestine, 17
    Galen on, 57
    obstructions into, 40
intuition, van Helmont on, 70–72
intussusception, 30
irritability, Glisson's theory of, 131
Isaac, 243
Isidore, Bishop of Seville, 233

Jacob, 243
Jake the Janitor, 167–68, 205